Beauty
and the
East

Beauty
and the East

A BOOK OF
ORIENTAL BODY CARE

WENDY BUONAVENTURA

ILLUSTRATIONS BY ISOBEL EADY

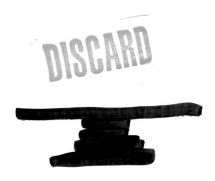

Interlink Books

An imprint of Interlink Publishing Group, Inc.
New York • Northampton

First American edition published 2001 by

INTERLINK BOOKS
An imprint of Interlink Publishing Group, Inc.
99 Seventh Avenue • Brooklyn, New York 11215 and
46 Crosby Street • Northampton, Massachusetts 01060
www.interlinkbooks.com

Text copyright © Wendy Buonaventura 1998, 2001
Illustrations copyright © Isobel Eady 1998, 2001

Originally published in Great Britain by Saqi Books

ISBN 1-56656-387-9

Printed and bound in Korea

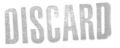

To request our complete 48-page full-color catalog, please call us toll free at **1-800-238-LINK,** visit our website at **www.interlinkbooks.com**, or write to
Interlink Publishing
46 Crosby Street, Northampton, MA 01060
e-mail: sales@interlinkbooks.com

Contents

Introduction

Beauty is all in the loving eye.
(Omar of Makhzum-Koraish)

I have a small block of amber which I keep in a pot by the side of my bed. And though it was many years ago that I bought it in a souk in Marrakesh, its fragrance is as fresh as if it were only yesterday. When I rub it on my arm and inhale its scent, it brings to mind the aroma of the spice markets: the sweet smell of sandalwood and cedarwood shavings in the wood-carvers' market and the rosewater perfume of the women as they brush past in the narrow alleys. On winter days at home when the air smells of soot and damp and traffic fumes, I lift the lid of my amber pot and I am straightaway transported to the spice souks of North Africa.

This is a book about the pleasures of the senses, about things we can do to make ourselves feel well-cared-for and sensually alive. The customs described in these pages come from Africa, Asia and the Middle East, and if there is one feature which they all have in common it is fragrance. Flowers, spices and perfumed oils are used in abundance in the East. Apart from cleansing and scenting the body, they are used to flavour food, to give clothes a delicate perfume, to scent furniture and hangings and in the ritual grace-notes of hospitality which are part of everyday life.

In ancient Egypt the first duty towards guests was to perfume their wigs with scented oils and adorn them with garlands of flowers. Pharaonic frescos of banquet scenes show women wearing tall tallow cones impregnated with perfumed wax on their heads. During the course of the evening this wax would melt with the heat, sending trickles of aromatic scent through their hair. This is one custom which I have not yet tried. But there are many others described in this book which I have sampled and found delightful, especially those involving a group, which inevitably lead to a party!

In many non-industrial cultures, where men and women spend much of their time apart, everyday activities tend to become group activities, and this is especially true of washing and grooming. In the West on the other hand most of our body care, apart from going to the hairdresser, is intensely private. It's also hurried. We're not used to indulging ourselves (that pejorative word!) by spending hours steaming ourselves clean. Whenever I go to a Turkish bath in Europe, I always notice that there is someone who looks slightly embarrassed and is perhaps perched uneasily on the very edge of the tub with her knees clamped together, trying to read a book. Some women stay as short a time as possible and regard a trip to the baths as being no more than a routine cleansing session; they don't see it as an opportunity for an evening of relaxing, unwinding and socializing. But if you want to derive the most pleasure from the baths then all of these are aspects of the experience.

In the Middle East and North Africa a visit to the hammam (Turkish bath) once consumed the entire day, and among the wealthy it was an excuse for a party, with female dancers and musicians brought in to entertain. Today, the modernization and increasing homogeneity of cultures the world over, plus the fact that more people have a bathroom in their homes, have led to the gradual disappearance of the hammam in the Middle East. Certainly the wealthier members of society no longer use the public baths. But the hammam is still widely used in countries like Morocco, where the best aspects of traditional women's culture have been retained, including that of painting intricate designs on the body with henna.

The steam bath was always an aspect of city rather than rural life, and it was a place for more than simple bodily cleansing. One of the final rituals of the day was the application of make-up, which had a magical, protective element attached to it. Indeed, many superstitions are still associated with the use of cosmetics today; for body care and hospitality are partly to do with protection against psychic forces and the intangible realm of the spirits.

They are also to do with identity and self-respect. Throughout history, women the world over have used their bodies to affirm their identity. For thousands of years women have resorted to the most ingenious, even bizarre methods of taking care of themselves and enhancing their charms.

When I browse through books about health and body care, however, I am often struck by an underlying tone of masochism, as though self-denial and pain were the path to well-being. So alongside all the innumerable articles and programmes about the pleasures of food, we have anorexia and bulimia and a highly profitable (for some) diet business.

We also have a multi-million-pound beauty industry dominated by men and dedicated to fostering false needs and insecurity in us. The beauty business is expert at persuading us to waste our money on expensive products with inflated claims of what they can do for us.

But we don't have to spend a small fortune on cleansers and cosmetics. There are simple beauty remedies that we can easily make for ourselves and which are every bit as effective as those we find in the shops. None of them involve hours of laborious preparation. (Who, these days, is willing to make time for such things, when it is so easy to go out and buy a ready-made product?) These alternative remedies use fruit, vegetables, olive oil, lemons and similar ingredients which we are more than likely to have in the kitchen cupboard. And it is satisfying to know that we are using fresh ingredients rather than chemicals on our bodies; that we can look after our hair and skin without having to buy wastefully packaged products whose ingredients are worth a fraction of their cost.

Apart from being good at persuading us to invest in overpriced cosmetics, the beauty business has succeeded in imposing on us a highly limiting concept of beauty. But if there is one thing we learn from looking at the female ideal in different cultures, it is that it differs widely from country to country. Among the Toposa tribe of Africa, women whose front teeth stick out are highly valued for their resemblance to cows, which are high-status animals in Toposa culture. On the other hand, the Baluba women of the Congo knock out their front teeth and file those which remain to a fine point as part of their cosmetic tradition.

Altering our bodies in small ways to conform to a cultural stereotype is nothing new, of course, and neither is plastic surgery. Two hundred years ago the Duchess of Marlborough, a well-known beauty, decided she would like to have a Grecian profile. Wax was injected into the hollow bridge of her nose, which gave her the sought-after straight line running from her forehead to the tip of her nose, and the operation was considered a great success. Until, that is, the Duchess took a summer holiday in the south of France. There, in the hot sun, the wax melted and trickled down beneath her skin until it formed two turkey-wattles which hung pendulously from her chin as a permanent reminder of her folly.

If this sounds horrifying, it is surely no worse than having silicone injected into our body or having the top layers of our skin removed by dermabrasion (by all accounts, a horribly painful procedure) in the hope that it will make us look twenty years younger. Throughout the world, irrational beliefs and culturally induced fears lead women to mutilate their bodies and subject them to all kinds of painful processes in a desperate desire to match up to other people's ideas of how they should look. And it is ironic to think that a physical characteristic which, in the West, may be thought disfiguring may be considered highly desirable elsewhere.

In a certain part of Indonesia, birth defects such as a club foot or twisted arm are considered the height of beauty. In Gabon, West Africa, large feet are prized above all other physical characteristics, while in Papua New Guinea, firm breasts are thought ugly and mothers pull their adolescent daughters' breasts in order to achieve the dangling effect which is considered a prerequisite for attracting a husband. One of the most horrific traditions undergone in order to satisfy cultural mores is that of the Padong women of northern Thailand. As 9-year-old girls they are fitted with the first of a number of brass collars, with one more added each year until they marry. These closely fitting brass rings elongate their necks, and if removed, the women would not be able to hold their heads up, so completely have their neck muscles atrophied over the years.

The only constant factor in all of this seems to be the punishing extremes to which women are prepared to go, and the pain they are prepared to suffer, in order to satisfy their society's ideal of female beauty.

Today's fashion designers have persuaded millions of women that volup-tuousness is gross, that we should have boys' bottoms and that the haggard faces of starving schoolgirls are attractive. But this wasn't always the case. In Britain, from Elizabethan to Edwardian times, a well-filled-out bottom was *de rigueur*. Beneath their skirts, less well-endowed women wore bum-rolls and farthingales to draw attention to their bottoms and achieve what stage-door Johnnies called 'the meat in the seat'. The fashion for skirts pulled tight in the front and swept up in a bustle at the back was praised in 1858 by the French writer Théophile Gautier as providing 'a pedestal for the bosom and head'. For hundreds of years artists have celebrated female flesh. As late as the 1950s no woman fretted if she had curves like Marilyn Monroe, who, in a 1990s poll of the woman most people would like to meet, came second.

In non-industrial countries weight is traditionally a sign of status, the supreme reflection of wealth and a leisured lifestyle. It is also considered the height of beauty. In the Arab world, a woman who could swing and shake her bottom from side to side in an alluring fashion when walking or dancing was awarded the highest praise. As Salahaddin al-Munajjid wrote: 'The cannons of female beauty require voluminous buttocks. The behind has to be tender and supple. It has been compared with a sand-dune on account of its height and softness and also to a sandy hill.'

In ancient Arabic poetry, comparing a woman to the sun or moon was highly complimentary. In Djerba (Tunisia) a future bride used to be locked away for months on end and fattened up like a goose; she was only allowed to emerge when her family felt she was sufficiently plump. This force-feeding was finally outlawed, after a great deal of publicity, by President Bourguiba. But if we go back several hundred years to the period of the Umayyads and the Abbasids, we find a more streamlined image popular in the Arab world. Breasts just big enough to be held in the palm of the hand were greatly appreciated; even a flat chest was prized for its novelty value, as well as a slim waist and a boyish bottom. Today, with the increasing domination of Western aesthetics throughout the world, and certainly among expatriate Arabs, the plump, motherly ideal no longer holds sway. Even so, and despite what the fashion industry would have us believe, it is not only in the Arab world that men secretly like to see a plump, shapely rump on a woman.

Bold, saucy movements of the bottom and swaying, sinuous hips are the focus of Arab women's dance. It is a dance which women perform in private for their own amusement, and though it is not practised in order to keep fit, one of its side-effects is that it helps keep the body supple and well toned. And who would deny that keeping in shape by dancing is a delightful alternative to a soulless exercise routine or a grim weight-watching diet?

It was through Arabic dance that I first encountered many of the customs described in this book. My work as a dancer opened the door to another culture: its music, poetry and food, its legendary hospitality and its traditions of female body care. I have delightful memories of eating oranges with friends in the steam bath, of sitting out in the sun having my feet painted with delicate henna designs, and of so much else besides. I hope that anyone who reads this book will be tempted to try some of the customs described in its pages, and in doing so will share the same thrill of discovery as when I first encountered them.

1

A Day at the Baths

Then she raised her garments to her neck and she looked like a
silver reed, illuminated with golden water . . . below her slim waist
there quivered a swaying bottom and a rounded navel so beautiful
that my fantasy cannot describe it . . .

(Anonymous fourteenth-century Arab text)

One afternoon in the 1970s I went to a hammam in Istanbul. It was my first experience of a Turkish bath and I think I was the only tourist there that day. Some of the women sat waiting for a scrub-down from the old washerwoman at the huge marble slab in the middle. We sat soaping ourselves at marble basins in the dim, echoing hall, swathed in clouds of vapour. High above our heads shafts of light fell from the dome through tiny windows cut in the shape of stars. There was a tremendous racket going on, the women's voices bouncing off the walls as they gossiped and exchanged news from one end of the hall to the other.

Slowly my eyes grew accustomed to peering through the steamy air and I surveyed the scene with interest. All around me women sat vigorously scrubbing themselves and their friends with rough woollen cloths. Some of them had the butts of soggy cigarettes stuck in the corners of their mouths, though this didn't prevent them from carrying on talking and at the same time using both hands to wash their friends' hair.

Suddenly I realized with horror that I was the only woman there who was entirely nude. Everyone else was wearing knee-length white bloomers saturated with steam. When they noticed my nudity a heated discussion sprang up. Some of the women began pointing at me and I thought to myself, surely it's too late to correct my *faux pas* – better to sit it out. But when my presence continued to be the main focus of attention I turned to a middle-aged Frenchwoman at the basin next to mine and asked if I should leave.

'It doesn't matter,' she shrugged. She was clearly a regular, for she called out casually to the old washerwoman, who wore a loincloth loosely fastened round her waist. When the Frenchwoman said a few words to her, she looked me up and down and gave a cackle of mirth. Then, lifting her arms above her head, she began singing and rolling her hips. When she tried to drag me to my feet to dance with her I felt like grabbing my towel and fleeing – I'm glad I didn't, as otherwise I'd probably never have ventured back and I'd have missed an extraordinary experience.

My enduring memory of that first steam bath is of being led to the marble slab where the old woman proceeded to subject me to the full range of her skills. She dipped her hand in a tub of olive-oil soap as thick and dark as honey and scooped out a handful. She rubbed it all over my body, smoothing it in with strong, experienced fingers. Then she scrubbed me with a rough woollen cloth and sluiced me down with pails of tepid water. Thinking she was done, I was about to lever myself upright when I felt her bony fingers sink into the muscles on either side of my shoulder-blades. She pummelled and kneaded and rolled me as if I were a lump of meat on a butcher's block. Then she slapped me sharply all over, as if tenderizing a fillet of steak, tossed one last pail of water over me and I was dismissed.

Compared to the hasty showers and baths I was used to, the steam bath was a revelation. Left to myself to recover, I lay down and closed my eyes, wrapped in a moist, all-embracing warmth like that of a tropical beach. I had the sensation of being as clean as a newborn baby, and when I ran my finger over my arm it felt like satin and my skin gave a little squeak of thanks.

For those of us who live in a cold climate it's difficult to relax and unwind completely. Heat is the greatest aid to relaxation and a steam bath or sauna is one of the few places where we're warm enough to really let go. The bath is also one place where we feel we can justifiably lie back and do absolutely nothing. At home there's always something we feel we should be doing. The odd little bit of free time we manage to snatch in our lives is likely to be interrupted by the phone or doorbell ringing, and many of us think we have to use every minute of our time following active pursuits. Not many of us feel that doing nothing is acceptable.

But just doing nothing in a pleasurable environment is pure bliss! A Caribbean woman who regularly goes to the nineteenth-century Turkish bath in Harrogate told me: 'The world out there demands so much of women these days. I think it's important that we look after ourselves, physically and mentally. And there aren't many places where women can be with other women in a protective environment, where you can take your clothes off and wander about and not feel vulnerable. That's why I go to the baths. You just lie there and let the heat work on your brain, and you rise above everything that's going on in your life.'

Another woman said: 'I love the sound of the water. I love the feeling of stripping away the world when I come in here. No husband, no family making demands on you.' Other women compared it to meditation, to a feeling of being on holiday. One of them said: 'What I like is that people aren't worried about what their bodies look like. You're all wandering around with nothing on and no one feels they have to meet some artificial standard of how to look. No one feels inhibited because they aren't perfect.'

Her friend commented: 'You realize, coming here, how you never quite relax, even when you think you do. Even when you're doing something like watching television, your mind's still racing and you're being bombarded by what's happening on the screen. Often quite disturbing things, too. There's so much pressure at work, so much pressure everywhere, so many things hitting at you. It's really important for my sanity, coming to the baths.'

But the last word must go to a Yorkshire woman for whom it takes three hours to reach the Harrogate baths and who says it's worth every minute of the arduous journey: 'It's your time to lie peacefully in the heat. It doesn't engage your thoughts. It's purely physical. It makes you feel like an animal! It's a pleasure you can't describe to anyone. You just have to experience it for yourself.'

A BRIEF HISTORY OF THE STEAM BATH

Benches covered with rugs followed the outline of the walls,
and sitting upon them, chattering like sparrows, we undressed
ourselves. Lengths of striped silk were given us, and tying them
about our hips we went into the next room, where walls of heated
stone surrounded a pool of warm water. We sat on the edge of the
pool and dabbled our toes in it while the bathers let down our
hair. Then we passed into the next room, as large as a mosque.

Lounging on carpeted slabs under the rays of the sun,
golden and green and red, that pierced the coloured glass
of the dome, we let the hours of the day trickle between our
idle fingers.

(Armen Ohanian, *The Dancer of Shamahka*)

It is assumed that people used perfumes liberally in the past to cover the more pungent smells of dirt and sweat. There may well be something in this; but in many countries attention to personal cleanliness is a requirement of religion as well as an aspect of well-being.

We read that in the ancient world people washed only their hands, feet and faces. Egypt alone was the exception. There, people washed their entire body daily and in some cases following every meal. In the houses of the wealthy, primitive showers have been excavated consisting of a large stone slab raised above the floor beside a drain. Here the bather would stand while being doused with water by a servant.

In the desert it remains the custom to give the body a brisk rub-down with sand. Soap was introduced from Mesopotamia (modern Iraq); made from soda or potash mixed with oil or clay, it was effective in dissolving dirt but was also unfortunately irritating to the skin. To counteract this abrasive effect, early moisturizers in the form of soothing oils and unguents were developed.

In countries where water is scarce, personal hygiene is often based on methods of cleansing which require little of this valuable resource. It is still common in such countries for women to 'wash' by subjecting the body to aromatic smoke.

In Sudan an earthenware pot filled with burning charcoal is placed in a hole dug in the sand. Pungent woods and resins are thrown into this pot – a combination of ginger, cloves, cinnamon, frankincense, sandalwood and myrrh. Then, wearing only her outer garment, a woman will crouch down in the hole with her cloak spread out all around her to trap the fumes. In this 'steam bath' the pores open and the body sweats out dirt and other impurities. On a visit to Sudan a friend of mine took part in this procedure. She told me that the heat is intense. And though the Sudanese women were accustomed to sitting in this steam bath for anything up to an hour, after only a few minutes my friend felt as if she was suffocating and begged to be allowed out!

Elaborate and pleasurable customs connected with personal hygiene developed with the introduction of the steam bath (called *hammam* in Arabic and *andaroon* in Farsi, or Persian). The steam bath developed out of Byzantine baths and

Roman thermae and spread rapidly during the period of Islamic expansion. Unlike the thermae, which were found only in big cities, the Middle Eastern hammam was widespread and was a feature of life in most small towns and villages. Tenth-century Baghdad had 27,000 hammams while in Cordoba (which, like the whole of Andalusia at that time, was under Muslim rule) there were between 5,000 and 6,000 of these establishments.

In the royal baths at the Topkapi Palace in Istanbul, women poured water from the white marble fountains over their bodies with gold and silver ladles. The relaxation rooms were splendidly carpeted and the divans covered in patterned silks. Evliya Çelebi Efendi, who visited the private bath of an Ottoman sultan in 1635, reported that the floors were covered in mosaics, the walls were scented with rosewater, musk and amber, and incense was kept constantly burning. The hammam was thought to be the favourite lurking place of spirits, both good (*jinn*) and bad (*afreet*), and incense was burned in the entrance as one of many protective rituals.

In the baths at the Alhambra, the most beautiful Islamic monument in all Andalusia, there was a balcony for the musicians who (so popular legend had it) were blind and therefore unable to spy on the ruler and his family at their ablutions.

Although the Islamic world took the idea of the steam bath from the Romans, their establishments were different in many ways. For one thing, Muslim men and women visited on different days of the week whereas men and women mixed freely in the Roman baths. In ancient Rome, a visit was often preceded by sporting activities and gymnasia, shops, libraries and even museums were attached to the bath complex. The baths of Caracalla were thought to be the most splendid of all ancient bath-houses. There Roman citizens had over two dozen mineral, steam, massage, friction and oil baths to chose from and vied with one another to find the most unusual fragrances to use in them.

In Islamic countries the emphasis was on purification and beautification rather than athleticism. Someone entering the hammam was considered to be full of impurities, and therefore weak and open to danger from the evil spirits which were thought to lurk in standing water to tempt bathers. The hammam was considered a particularly favourite haunt of both good and evil spirits, and in the past women took the precaution of uttering a prayer as they stepped across the threshold, entering the baths with the left foot and leaving later on with the right.

Unlike the thermae, the hammam was situated underground, with the water centrally heated beneath the floor. Visitors descended into the bowels of the earth to enjoy the offerings of the various rooms in an atmosphere of womb-like warmth and comfort. Masseurs, hairdressers (who also practised various forms of medicine), herbalists and magicians all plied their trades at the baths, as well as attendants who gave clients a good soaping following by a vigorous pummelling. Julia Pardoe, who visited a Turkish bath in the late nineteenth century, commented on the appearance of these women:

> From constantly living in a sulphurous atmosphere, their skins have become of the colour of tobacco, and of the consistency of parchment; many among them were elderly women, but not one of them was wrinkled; they had, apparently, become aged like frosted apples.

In a well-appointed steam bath different rooms are set aside for different activities. There are rooms of varying degrees of heat for sweating out the dirt, hot and cold showers and swimming pools filled with warm and cold water. When describing the main hall of a pasha's steam bath, Pardoe commented on the projecting galleries surrounding it on all sides, rather like boxes in a theatre, which were richly furnished with cushions, mattresses and rugs. There, to the soothing tinkling of fountains in the background, women relaxed after the rigours of the day's activities, wearing white linen robes embroidered and fringed with gold, while attendants dressed their hair. A wealthy woman might have five different costumes taken to the baths for her to change into, each wrapped in a silk bundle embroidered with pearls. The servants also transported mattresses, brass basins, food, drink and all the other paraphernalia needed for the day.

Of course, not all hammams were places of splendour. And the customs written about by Western orientalists related only to the lives of the rich. These writers did not report on the lives of the poor, but even poor women gave themselves treats like henna decoration. Certainly, cleanliness has never been a prerogative of the wealthy in Arab society, but is an important aspect of the Islamic faith. One hammam that I visited in a south Moroccan village consisted of a single chamber with a hole cut in the domed roof. Through this hole a dusty pillar of sunlight illuminated the shadowy cavern with its uneven flagstones and dripping brown earthen walls.

In the past a visit to the baths was a leisurely business, with every possible shred of enjoyment wrung from the occasion. For women confined to the harem most of the time, the hammam was above all a place to socialize and pick up news and gossip of the outside world. As Pardoe recorded:

> The centre of the floor is like a fair; sweet-meat, sherbet and fruit merchants parade up and down, hawking their wares. Negresses pass to and fro with the dinners or chibuks [pipes] of their several mistresses; secrets are whispered, confidences are made; and together, the scene is so strange, so new, and withal so attractive, that no European can fail to be interested.

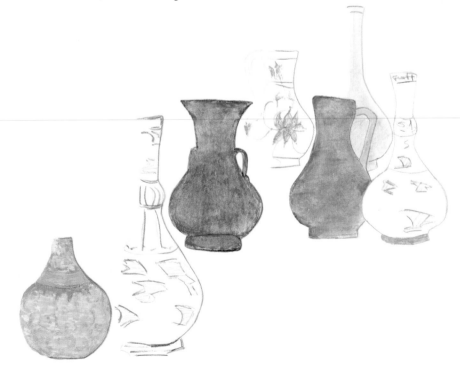

Isabel Burton, a contemporary of Pardoe, is another traveller who left a detailed account of a day at the baths in Istanbul. After undressing, she wrapped herself in a length of silk, with a towel wound round her head to counteract the effect of the heat. On returning to England, she visited one of the newly opened Turkish baths in London. She records coming to the aid of a fellow bather, an English-woman who had taken none of the normal precautions and, having turned as red as a lobster, was on the verge of fainting when Burton found her. (She promptly picked up a towel, dipped it in cold water and wound it round the woman's head.) In her memoirs she notes that the atmosphere in the London baths was sadly lacking in the gaiety and delight of the Istanbul baths, where after receiving a massage she made her way to the retiring room. She fell asleep surrounded by women smoking the narghile (hubble-bubble pipe) and reclining with cups of bitter coffee. She records how delightful it was waking up to the sound of music and the sight of young girls dancing and chasing each other across the flower-strewn floor.

In societies where women spend most of their time together they tend to develop a close physical ease with one another. Nineteenth-century accounts of the Turkish baths did much to create the outsider's image of Middle Eastern women as leading lives of indolent, even flagrant, sensuality. The communal bathing habits of the Middle East were something of an affront to middle-class ladies like Pardoe. Between the lines of her and other travellers' accounts we sense that they found aspects of the experience, however fascinating, rather too much for their delicate sensibilities:

> The heavy, dense, sulphurous vapour that filled the place and almost suffocated me – the wild, shrill cries of the slaves pealing through the reverberating domes of the bathing halls, enough to awaken the very marble with which they were lined – the subdued laughter and whispered conversation of their mistresses – the sight of nearly three hundred women, only partially dressed, and that in fine linen so perfectly saturated with vapour that it revealed the whole outline of the figure – the busy slaves passing and repassing, naked from the waist upwards, and with their arms folded upon their bosoms,

balancing on their heads piles of fringed or embroidered napkins – groups of lovely girls laughing, chatting and refreshing themselves with sweetmeats, sherbets and lemonade – parties of playful children, apparently quite indifferent to the dense atmosphere which made me struggle for breath and, to crown all, the sudden bursting forth of a chorus of voices into one of the wildest and shrillest of Turkish melodies, that was caught up and flung back by the echoes of the vast hall … all combined to form a picture like the illusory semblance of a phantasmagoria, almost leaving me in doubt whether that on which I looked were indeed reality, or the mere creation of a distempered brain.

The hammam was a popular subject of orientalist art. Painters created the image of fleshly female indulgence with vistas of perfectly formed, pale-skinned nude women. But most of these artists were men and they would not have been admitted to the baths on women's day. It is unlikely that the women were completely nude; accounts describe them wearing lengths of fabric knotted round their hips, or shifts of finest muslin, with high wooden pattens on their feet. These pattens protected the bathers from the heated marble and stopped them slipping on floors swimming with soapsuds and water. The plainest pattens were made of walnut, with leather straps to secure them. More expensive ones were of rosewood, ebony and sandalwood inlaid with tortoiseshell and mother-of-pearl. The costliest ones of all were studded with turquoise and pearls.

Orientalists are sometimes criticized for giving a false impression of a complex culture by concentrating only on the sensuality of the women's lives. But, as a Lebanese friend of mine observed: 'Why shouldn't a woman be sensuous if she is also independent and strong? I'm afraid this is a sort of austere protestant image that has even been entering the Arab world recently. You find some Arabs now being ashamed of images of the sensuous East, all the beautiful things, the perfumes and fabrics, the dancing. But one of the positive aspects of Arab culture is that these things were never separated in the past; they were all part of life to be enjoyed.'

WESTERN ATTITUDES TO BATHING

Hippocrates, the father of medicine, recommended a daily bath and massage with essential oils to maintain a healthy body. The ancient Greeks and Romans were among the world's most enthusiastic bathers, but the further north we travel, the more suspicious people are about the idea of immersing the body in water. In medieval England it was thought that the delicate balance of the body's four 'humours' would be upset by exposing it to water. Besides, washing was associated with pagan practices. As far back as the days of the Crusades, men returning from war in the Holy Land tried to establish the steam bath in Europe. But these establishments rapidly degenerated into places of low repute and were consequently closed down. Total immersion in water, even the most perfunctory washing, was not popular in Europe until relatively recently and was unknown in Europe before the seventeenth century, though Queen Elizabeth I commented that she took a bath once a month, whether she needed it or not!

It is difficult for us today to imagine the stench of people's bodies a couple of hundred years ago. And perhaps it isn't surprising that people distrusted water and thought that too much exposure to it would damage their health. In the eighteenth century, London's water supplies were primitive. Most people relied on water taken from the River Thames, which was contaminated with sewage. For many, soap was expensive and beyond their reach; so not only did people's bodies reek, their clothes were positively rancid. Even the wealthy were filthy. Their wigs crawled with lice, some had mice nesting in their hair, and women carried antiseptic pouches in their bodices to kill the bugs which fell out of their hair. Women's gowns trailed in the dirt of unpaved streets, picking up traces of the sewage in which everyone trod as a matter of course. The rich spent a great deal of money on perfume, especially civet and musk, to mask the dreadful stench of their bodies, and toilet water was liberally used to this end; but visitors from the East nonetheless continued to comment on the terrible smell at social gatherings in the capitals of Europe.

It is only relatively recently that Europeans have begun to lose their distrust of immersion in water, and that improved water supplies have brought cleanliness within the reach of the majority of the population in their own homes. In Scandinavia, though, there is a long tradition of steam-cleansing; the sauna had a ritual importance as a meeting-place and was also the place where women gave birth.

THE STEAM BATHS AND ISLAM

An Algerian woman who recently came to live in England was delighted when she discovered the old Turkish bath in the city of Harrogate. 'We decided to choose a country where our life would be less restricted,' she told me. 'We were living under religious pressure which prohibited women from showing themselves in any public place without wearing the *hijab* (veil). My mother-in-law, who is Muslim, suddenly decided that Islam is against women going to the baths because the women watch each other and we start thinking about sex.'

Her Caribbean friend laughed. 'Well, when you're so clean, that's the time you do feel sexual. You feel so clean, so alive, from your head right down to your toes, that when you go home you do feel sexy!'

The Algerian woman went on: 'I told my mother that all this business about women looking at each other was a male conspiracy, because men know that the only freedom left to women in Algeria is going to the bath! It's the only place we can go by ourselves. My mother, for example, didn't go out very much. She needed a good reason to do so. Going to the hammam wasn't a problem in the past. I think men want to find an excuse to stop us enjoying ourselves. So they invent this business about sexy looks as a way to stop us going out.'

Muslim writers have written about the hammam as a place of great eroticism. Cultures that are intent on maintaining strict control of female sensuality continue to thunder against nudity in the baths and exhort women to cover their bodies even in the presence of other women. But as Tunisian sociologist Abdelwahab Bouhdiba comments in his book *Sexuality in Islam*, the creation of the hammam has given Muslim society:

a valuable instrument for itself to channel the sexual drives liberated by religion, but repressed by the misogynist puritanism that grew up over the centuries and by a strict, universal separation of the sexes that might have proved fatal to it.

Unlike Judaism and Christianity, from which the Muslim faith drew much of its initial inspiration, Islam is alone in celebrating the pleasures of the senses in its religious literature. Nevertheless, according to orthodox thought, the hammam is a dangerous place of temptation. Right down to the present day, writers of a fundamentalist persuasion have not only exhorted women to keep their bodies covered in the baths, but have discouraged them from even going there in the first place.

Ironically, it is in the hammam that Muslim boys first learn about women's bodies. For male children do not accompany their fathers to the hammam, they go with their mothers until they reach puberty. The female attendant at the baths keeps a strict eye open and the day inevitably comes when she notices that a young boy is looking at the women around him with rather too much interest. 'From now on,' she will say to his mother, 'let him come here with his father.'

The elaborate rituals of cleanliness, the sugaring and the application of henna, far from being part of a mysterious female world, are witnessed by boys at a very young age. In the Qur'an's sumptuous images of paradise, the male imagination has recreated the remembered pleasures of the steam bath, with its atmosphere of enveloping warmth and femininity. But the familiarity with women's nude bodies which, unlike their Western counterparts, Muslim boys enjoy in early life, comes to an abrupt end when the first signs of puberty appear. From that day onward, the door to the women's world is closed to them. In future the young boy will have little contact with the female half of humanity – even the women in his own family become strangers to some degree.

Bouhdiba describes the hammam as a mythical, womblike place full of the mysteries of femininity, which becomes almost a subject of revenge to the males who have been so rudely thrust out of it. At puberty, he writes:

The gap between the sexes . . . is now consummated . . . The world of women is a 'sub-world', devoid of seriousness and all too easily treated with the contempt that boosts the male's confidence in himself, in his knowledge, in his wishes and in his power.

Having grown up with a more intimate knowledge of women and their private world than Western boys, the sense of exclusion is severe. From now on men will only ever revisit this private world in memory and in the dreams of a mythical paradise, whose principal delight lies in the presence of beautiful, compliant women and in the relaxed, open closeness between the sexes which, according to the Qur'an, is a feature of life in paradise but which is far from being an aspect of earthly life in Islamic society.

Roses

*I said that when I reached the
rose garden I would pick an armful
of blooms to give to my friends.
But when I did reach it the perfume
of the rose made me so drunk that
I forgot my promise.*

(Sheikh Saadi of Shiraz)

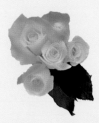 No flower has been the subject of more descriptions and poems than the rose. It was the Persians who cultivated the art of making exquisite pleasure gardens and developed the preservation of flowers. One of the most beautiful of all Persian classical poems, the *Gulistan* [Rose Garden] by Sheikh Saadi of Shiraz, was composed in praise of the red rose. It is said that he wrote it after spending the night in his garden with a friend. In the

morning his companion plucked some roses and placed them among the folds of his clothes, to perfume them with their fragrance. Saadi told his friend to throw the flowers away, adding that they would only live for one day, whereas he was going to write a poem about the rose garden which would last for all eternity. Today it remains one of the most popular of all Persian poems.

In Syria (a name which, according to some sources, derives from *suri*, meaning 'land of roses'), the flower is grown in nearly every garden. Damascus is still well known for its cultivation of the damask rose, which lent its name to the town and to the damask silk made there in the colour of this flower.

In the fourteenth and fifteenth centuries the Crusaders took home with them a liking for rose toilet water, or 'damask water' as they called it.

A favourite massage oil of Indian women, *urgujja*, is composed chiefly of attar of rose and essence of jasmine – the two most expensive essential oils. Today Morocco is the largest producer of rose oil. The flowers are gathered at dawn in the late spring while the petals are still wet with dew (as the sun rises, the essential oil content of the flowers rapidly falls) and are immediately sent to be distilled. It takes thirty roses to produce a single drop of oil, and because of this low yield, rose remains one of the most costly essential oils: fifty times more expensive than others. The distilled oil has a by-product, an attar which rises to the top and is collected and left to solidify. A seventeenth-century traveller to Persia wrote that attar of roses 'is more valuable than gold, and nothing in the world possesses a perfume so agreeable and sweet'.

Today, intensive breeding of roses for their longevity and

bloom size has had the accidental side-effect of reducing their fragrance. Roses which we buy from the florist today are bigger, brighter and longer-lasting than those of ten years ago. But research suggests that the methods used to achieve this result have damaged the scent-producing properties of the flower. Cells which generate scent in rose petals also make the flowers wilt more quickly; petals with large numbers of these cells, and hence a more potent scent, are thinner and weaker and are quicker to drop off.

Rose essence, which has a healing effect on the liver, was used in the past to flavour wine; it was also thought to lessen the effects of alcohol and help prevent a hangover.

Rosewater is used as a face cleanser and is especially good for oily skin.

A concentrated syrup, made by boiling up rose petals and adding sugar, is a wonderfully refreshing drink, diluted and chilled with ice. As an alternative to this time-consuming process, you can buy bottles of concentrated rosewater from Middle Eastern and Asian grocery stores and dilute a little of this in water.

2

Cleansing

*Voluptuous women inflame the hearts of all men with their
lascivious graces; they chat with one man, dart provocative
glances at another and a third occupies their heart.*

(The *Kama Sutra*)

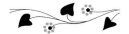

A number of Turkish baths built in Europe in the nineteenth century remain in
use today. Some of them have swimming pools, saunas and private cubicles with
starched sheets for relaxing in afterwards. The most enterprising offer refreshments and treatments such as massage, and some of them have become venues
for evening programmes of dance and exercise. Some of these establishments
try to make the experience as pleasurable as possible, with all kinds of nice little
touches, such as steam rooms scented with aromatic oil.

*Before you contemplate sampling the delights of a Turkish bath or sauna, you should
bear the following in mind:*

*A well-regulated bath shouldn't be so hot as to make you feel uncomfortable.
Even so, a few precautions are necessary. Steam baths and saunas stimulate the blood
supply to the skin and they also increase the pulse rate. So if you suffer from any
kind of heart problems, you MUST consult your doctor first.*

*Give yourself plenty of time. Don't imagine you can cram a visit to the baths into
an hour between work engagements. You won't get nearly as much out of it if you're
in a hurry; and you won't be able to relax completely unless you give yourself at
least a couple of hours, if not more. Afterwards you will probably be far too relaxed
to think of doing anything more taxing than lying on the sofa.*

Different days of the week are set aside for men and women, but some baths have one mixed-sex 'couples' day and one ordinary mixed-sex day each week. I wouldn't recommend going to a mixed-sex day alone, unless you fancy the idea of being a lone woman surrounded by the local rugby team. The big hotels which have health clubs often allow non-residents to use the facilities for a small fee; in this case the sauna and steam rooms are usually mixed and you are required to wear a swimsuit.

What To Take With You

It's a good idea to take a cool drink or some fruit to share. With a group of friends, a big bag of oranges soon disappears as well as creating a delicious fragrance.

You may also like to take a bottle of ordinary tap water containing a few drops of essential oil. When you enter the sauna you can pour this over the hot coals if nobody else minds. Eucalyptus and rosemary are both good for relieving colds and stuffiness. Or you can use olbas oil, which includes eucalyptus, menthol, peppermint, wintergreen, clove, cajuput and juniper.

Most Western baths provide lockers and towels as part of the entrance fee, and towelling robes at an extra cost. Some women take a swimsuit to wear, but it's much better for the body, and helps the sweating process, if you undress completely. You are likely to find soap, shampoo, tissues and a hairdryer in the changing-cum-shower area; but you may prefer to take your own favourite cleansers with you, as well as henna and any other treatments you intend giving yourself. Don't forget a loofah or scrubbing mitt.

The Bath Routine

It's always more enjoyable to go to the baths in a group and make a social occasion of it than to go alone. I sometimes notice a woman sitting on her own, looking rather tense and trying to read a book. I wouldn't recommend reading in the steam room as, apart from anything else, it will stop you relaxing, and one of the most pleasurable aspects of the experience lies in emptying your mind and opening up to the smells and sights and activities going on around you.

Sometimes, when women don't know the procedure they simply have a soapy shower, then sit in their towels for ten minutes, after which they decide that it's time

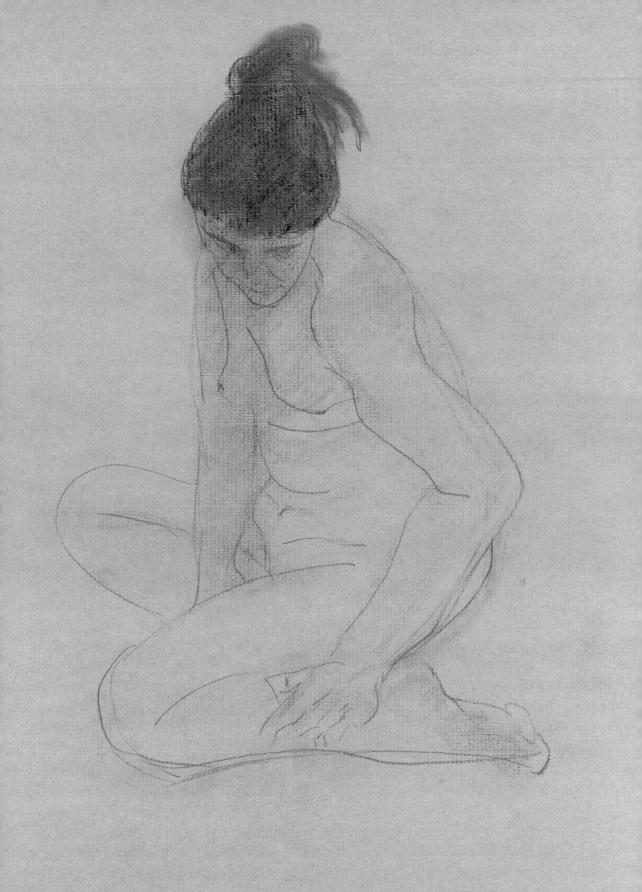

to go! So, for anyone who has never been to a steam bath, here is the routine:

Take a shower before entering the steam room or sauna. (A sauna has dry heat, as opposed to a Turkish steam room, which is vaporous. You may find one of these suits you better than the other.) A warm shower will open your pores and help the sweating process get going. It's customary not to use soap at this stage.

Prolonged exposure to steam is not good for the hair, so you may like to wrap your head in a cool, damp towel. If you are extra-sensitive to heat, this towel will also help keep you cool and it can be repeatedly renewed by damping it down with cold water.

Limit your first steam to 10 minutes. By then you will probably be feeling the need for a cool shower. The general procedure is to alternate steaming with a cold shower, which will bring down the body's temperature before further steaming. In a sauna, the lower benches are the coolest. If you want a more intense heat you will find a bucket of water which you can ladle onto the coals.

A Turkish bath generally has two or three rooms at progressively hotter temperatures, but there's no need to sit in all of them just to show how tough you are. Some Western steam baths have an outdoor hot tub and barrel sauna, and the most enterprising ones can be hired for private late-night celebrations.

Washing with soap comes after a thorough steaming. Either give yourself a good scrub with a loofah or rough woollen mitt or book a scrub-down (which may come with a vigorous massage).

Some women like to apply a face pack while they're having a steam; but you may choose to do this only after you've had a thorough scrubbing and cleansing.

A shampoo generally comes last, along with other optional treatments such as depilation and henna.

If you want a massage you will have to pre-book one as soon as you arrive at the baths. If you aren't having a massage, find your way to the relaxation room where you can recline in your towelling robe and get used to a cooler temperature in preparation for the outside world. Some baths provide magazines and games, most offer refreshments and some even have private cubicles furnished with little tables and lamps.

Lemons

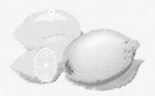

The versatile lemon can be put to many uses in body care, either alone or in combination with other foods. Lemon juice cleans and restores acidity to the skin; it is also antiseptic and helps prevent blemishes. It is a truly effective cleanser and is good for eliminating strong food smells like garlic and fish from the hands after cooking.

The ancient Egyptians used lemons as a shampoo to cut into the oil which made dirt cling to the hair. They rubbed lemon peel over the teeth and gums as a breath freshener and also used it to remove brown stains from the teeth.

Alone or mixed with rosewater, lemon is a good astringent. A little lemon juice added to a foot bath helps soften and relieve tired feet.

And if all these external uses were not enough, lemons are rich in vitamins D and C, which heal the skin and small blood vessels.

A little fresh lemon juice in hot water taken before breakfast is good for the digestive system.

A Lemon Exfoliant

Rub a light vegetable or nut oil over your face. Pat on a thin layer of warm water, then a layer of freshly squeezed lemon juice. After a minute or so, and before the oil or lemon juice has time to dry on the skin, rub this emulsion in a circular motion with the fingers over a small patch of skin until a little ball of it forms, which you can then discard. Continue this procedure over your entire face and neck, so that the top layer of dead skin cells is removed.

A Lemon Skin-whitener

Lemons are used as a mild bleach and to tone down freckles in societies which regard freckles as skin blemishes. For a fair skin, mix equal parts of lemon juice and either elder-flower or rosewater. Pat this lotion onto the face and allow it to dry for anything from 15 minutes to a couple of hours. Wash off with tepid water. Close the pores with an astringent and remember to apply oil or a nourishing cream, as all herbal and food bleachers tend to have a drying effect on the skin.

A Remedy for Softening Rough Elbows

For softening (and whitening) rough dark elbows, cut a lemon in half, gouge out a little of the flesh and sit with an elbow propped up in each half.

A Final Hair Rinse for Fair Hair

Use lemon juice on its own, or mixed with lime juice or vinegar. Rubbed into the scalp, it is said to help prevent hair loss.

A Remedy for Sore Throats

A well-known remedy for sore throats and colds is lemon and honey in hot water. Make sure you do not use boiling water, which will kill the vitamin C.

FACE AND HAND TREATMENTS FROM OLD PERSIA

A Daily Face Wash for Open Pores

Mix rosewater with a third the quantity of the juice of sour oranges (these can be found in Western shops specializing in Middle Eastern food).

A Face Wash for Dry Skin

Use equal proportions of distilled water or fresh milk, together with fresh melon juice.

Some Delicious Remedies for Softening the Skin

(a)   *Use equal parts of black cherries and grapes; mix the juice of the squashed fruit with rosewater and apply daily as a face wash.*

(b)   *Blanch poppy flowers, drain off the water and place the flowers on the skin straightaway.*

(c)   *Boil parsley in its own juice together with a few drops of water (this remedy is also said to help cure acne).*

(d)   *Mix equal proportions of watercress juice and honey; apply and allow to dry on the face before rinsing off.*

A Peeler and Exfoliant

In Iran you can still buy sephidob, *a white clay containing bone meal and animal fat. For use as an exfoliant, apply a thin film of oil to your skin, then moisten the* sephidob *with water and rub some into a rough bath cloth (which should be at least as rough as a loofah). For the face, simply rub some* sephidob *onto wet fingers and use it as an exfoliant twice a month.*

THE MOUTH

The Inky Mouth

O strange and lovely sight:
A smudge of ink, all staining
A luscious mouth, containing
The wine of sweet delight.

(al-Barraq)

The 'balm' mentioned in the Book of Genesis is thought to be a gum which comes from the bark of the *Pistacia lentiscus* shrub. Known as mastic, it allegedly hardens the skin and is still used today to strengthen teeth and gums. It is an ingredient of toothpaste and was once used as an ingredient of a male aphrodisiac, mixed with honey and oil.

Many substances which were chewed to sweeten the breath had euphoric side-effects and we may think that in the case of some of them, such as opium, the primary attraction may have been their intoxicant qualities.

The oldest recipes for ointments and cleansers date back to the second century BC and include breath fresheners made of myrrh mixed with mint. In Palestine and Arabia mastic was chewed to sweeten the breath. Orris root, cinnamon and sandalwood have all been used for the same purpose and Indian restaurants often provide a little dish of caraway seeds to nibble at the end of a meal. Caraway leaves a refreshing taste in the mouth, but other traditional mouth cleansers still in use are not so attractive. Indians who chew betel have red-stained mouths, which makes them look as if their teeth and gums are dripping with blood, and Indian pavements are dotted with the red stains of spat-out betel juice. Another Middle Eastern remedy for cleansing the breath is to chew sage and in the souks you can find small bundles of *swek*, another traditional cleanser. *Swek* is the outer layer of the walnut root and resembles cinnamon bark in appearance. Like betel, it turns the gums a brilliant red.

Teeth and Breath Fresheners

It has always struck me as odd that a product designed to guard against tooth decay should contain sugar. Some commercial brands of toothpaste are unbearably sweet and it's a refreshing change to try a home-made alternative.

One of the oldest and best toothpastes is a light salt and water paste. Salt is an antiseptic and gargling with salt water is a common remedy for sore throats. Salt removes nicotine and berry stains from the teeth and if you rub it into your gums it will help deter the dreaded plaque.

A more delicious alternative to salt is a fresh strawberry squashed in the mouth and rubbed against each tooth.

Indian yogis use a tongue scraper in the morning, drawing it from the back to the front of the tongue, to clean away the impurities which have accumulated overnight. As a substitute, use an inverted teaspoon.

An old remedy for bleeding gums is to boil up watercress and rinse the mouth with the resulting liquid.

Chewing raw parsley is a popular way to get rid of the smell of garlic on the breath and is used all around the Mediterranean and in the Middle East. When you sit down in a Lebanese restaurant you will often find that the waiter will place a plate of parsley and mint on your table for this purpose.

Peppermint tea, lavender water, clove tea and rosewater are effective mouth washes. They should all be kept in the fridge.

PERSIAN AND ARAB METHODS OF DEPILATION

An Iranian friend of mine who was brought up in the West told me that when her mother comes to visit she often scolds her for the hair under her arms. 'She told me I should never wear sleeveless dresses if I intend going on this way, because the hair under the arms is like pubic hair. She said it would give strangers rude thoughts about me, especially men!'

My friend is very unusual in not removing her underarm hair, for great importance is attached to depilation in Islamic countries. Outside the towns, it is still customary to remove every trace of hair from the body, including that of the pubis, and complete depilation is part of the elaborate cleansing ritual which a bride undergoes before her wedding. But today, younger, Westernized women are abandoning the custom of full depilation.

In many cultures hair has great sexual significance and is thought to possess magical powers. A completely hairless body is the body of a child, and in this respect complete depilation has an element of robbing a woman of something of her sexual power. Among the pre-wedding rites of Hasidic Jews it is customary for a woman to shave her head and wear a wig so that her natural hair cannot work spells on her husband. In the West we tend to restrict depilation to our legs and underarms, though some of us don't feel obliged even to go this far and most Italian women wouldn't dream of removing their underarm hair. Hundreds of years ago hair was removed from the body with a paste based on yellow arsenic.

Fortunately this method was superseded long ago by other, less dangerous ones. Another ancient Middle Eastern method of removing pubic hair involved the foul-smelling cedre, which dissolved the hair in much the same way as a modern commercial depilatory.

Taking the above into consideration, it seems strange that in Iran and Turkey a hint of a moustache is seen as a mark of beauty in a woman; but then, aesthetics have little to do with consistency.

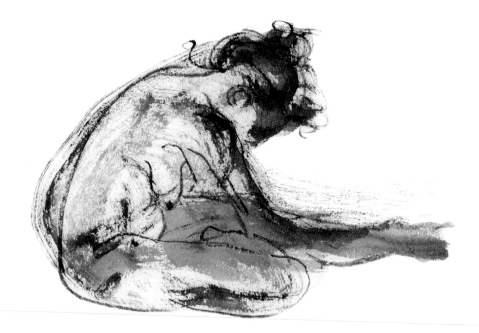

Band Andazi

Band andazi *is a Persian method of hair removal using strong cotton thread. The area to be depilated is given a light dusting of talcum powder. Then a length of thread is wound round the index and first fingers of both hands to make a loop, twisted in the middle (rather like a cat's cradle). By moving the thread swiftly over the area to be depilated, small groups of hairs are plucked out incredibly quickly: a professional* band andaz *can depilate one leg in three minutes! Sometimes you see these women with the thread draped round the neck or looped between the toes while working away with both hands, their bodies bobbing rhythmically backwards and forwards. A spot of wax is dabbed in the twisted part of the thread to prevent sticking. The hair needs to be dry for this method of depilation, so a professional* band andaz *will work at home rather than at the baths.*

Halawa or Sukkar

The most popular method of depilation throughout the Middle East and North Africa is *halawa*, or sugaring. Occasionally warmed beeswax is used but generally *halawa* is done with a mixture of lemon juice and sugar. It is a communal activity, with women taking it in turns to prepare the *sukkar* (sugar) solution for the group, and with several women around there is always someone to make sure it doesn't burn! Sometimes an expert is invited in to make the *sukkar*, and the *halawa* is followed up with a manicure.

A Lebanese friend recalled how, as a child, she and her friends used to watch their mothers making the caramel or sugaring solution, knowing that after it had been left to cool, all the children would be offered a small piece to eat: 'Our mothers used to get together once a month to do it, and it was a real treat for us, boys as well as girls. If it was a day for sugaring we'd beg our mothers: "Wait till we get home from school before you do it!" It was mesmerizing to see it being poured out of the pan, a beautiful golden colour. We had to wait until it was cool. A piece was sliced off for us and then we would be thrown out while our mothers got on with the serious work! There are some women who've made a successful business out of selling this *sukkar* ready-made in little pots. But even so, you can still find rich women sometimes saying: "Let's get together and make it ourselves", because it's fun.'

Nothing could be simpler and less expensive than to make up the sukkar *for yourself. Combine equal parts of sugar and lemon juice and add a pinch of salt (this is said to make the depilation process less painful). Stir this mixture constantly over a low heat until it begins to caramelize, bubbling and turning beige in colour. Remove from the heat and test by dropping a small globule into a glass of water. If it crystallizes it's ready; if not it needs further cooking. This is the only slightly difficult aspect of making the sugar solution: to bring it to the right consistency so that it's neither underdone nor burnt.*

When the solution is ready, pour it onto a marble slab or a lightly oiled tin tray and leave it to cool. You can make the mixture in large quantities and keep it in the freezer in small amounts, each in its own plastic bag. It can easily be reconstituted by suspending it, in its bag, over a dish of hot water.

When the sukkar *has cooled down, moisten your fingers, break off a piece and knead it as you would knead dough, stretching it to give it a pliable, elastic quality. Keep a wet cloth handy and if the* sukkar *starts to get dry and hard to handle, simply wet your fingers on the cloth and set to work again. Don't make the mistake of applying water directly to the* sukkar *or it will be ruined.*

Apply the mixture to the body by smoothing a strip downwards with the thumbs onto the area to be depilated. Pull it off straightaway with a brisk upwards movement (against the direction of hair growth), bringing the hair with it. You can use a single strip of sugar several times. If your skin is very sensitive and turns red, rub on a little neat lemon juice or a sprinkling of talcum powder.

After using this method for the first time the hair may grow back faster than usual, but it will be of a finer texture and gradually it will take longer to grow back.

DEAD SEA MUD

The quest for a soft, wrinkle-free complexion has led women to slap all kinds of animal and vegetable matter on their bodies over the years. Many a curious practice promising an eternally youthful skin has enjoyed its brief spell of popularity and we must assume that it wasn't mere whim which led Cleopatra to bathe in asses' milk. One of the more extreme practices, from a fourth-century Syrian book of medicine, recommended placing a camel's lung over the face. In ancient Rome, Nero's wife Poppaea set the fashion of going to bed in a mask made of perfumed bread paste. By dawn the mask had hardened and cracked, leaving her face looking like that of a wizened old hag! Soliman's Water, produced in Europe in the sixteenth century, was renowned for removing spots, freckles and warts, but this wasn't all it removed. Its main ingredient was sublimate of mercury, which stripped off the entire outer layer of skin. With continued use, it gradually corroded the flesh underneath and in the end a woman's teeth were likely to fall out too. A hundred years later, European women believed that by sleeping in a night mask made of silk, linen or even leather pulled tightly across the face, the lines would be smoothed out and eventually disappear altogether. But stretching and 'lifting' the skin in this way probably made it sag even further when it was released from its nightly corset.

We may laugh, but there are some ancient remedies based on folk wisdom which have now been awarded the scientific stamp of approval. A few years ago in Israel I went to an area of the Dead Sea which is surrounded by bare brown hills and desert stretching as far as the eye can see. Along this short patch of coastline men and women covered from head to toe in thick, glistening black mud were trooping down to the sea, where they lay bobbing up and down in the shallows. It was a strange sensation to be in water so salty it was impossible to either sink or swim in it, and when I attempted to lie back in the water and float, the water simply pushed me upright again, however hard I tried! After washing off the mud I had a dip in the warm sulphurous spring waters which feed the sea, and I was so exhausted afterwards that I fell asleep in the bus back to Jerusalem.

Dead Sea mud has been shown to contain many minerals and other constituents which feel as if they are sucking out all the impurities from the body. Nowadays you can find it in health food and body-care shops, so you don't need to go all the way to Israel to try it. But if you have the chance do take it, for it is an extraordinary experience.

Fair of Face

The desire for a golden tan is a recent phenomenon exclusive to the West. Historically a suntan marked you out as one of the poor, the working classes. A woman out toiling in the fields had no time to pamper her skin and shield it from the sun; thus a soft, milky complexion became the sign of a leisured lifestyle as well as a hallmark of beauty.

An ancient Assyrian skin bleach consisted of white lead mixed with egg white, which women used to leave on their faces overnight. This practice later spread to Europe via Greece and Rome and continued until the end of the eighteenth century, often resulting in disfigurement and death by poisoning.

A less drastic skin bleach was *batikha*. It was made by pounding cowrie shells with borax, white marble, rice, eggs and lemon together with a seed known as *helbas*. These ingredients were mixed inside a melon, with the addition of ground peas, beans, lentils and fruit pulp. The paste was then left out in the sun for a few days until it had dried and disintegrated into a fine white powder.

Today, in the personal columns of Indian newspapers, a woman who advertises herself as 'wheatish-complexioned' can expect to attract far more interest from potential husbands than her dark-skinned sisters; indeed, a dark skin is considered as great a handicap in the Indian marriage market as infertility, and may adversely affect the amount of a bride's dowry.

A widely practised pre-wedding treatment for an Indian bride uses a bright yellow paste of ground turmeric mixed with either milk, yoghurt or water and perfumed oil. This paste is rubbed all over the face, neck, arms and legs, right up to the thighs. Sometimes this procedure is followed for every one of the seven days preceding the wedding. The bride goes to bed covered in this paste, which is said to leave the skin silky soft and several degrees lighter in shade when it is washed off.

Olives

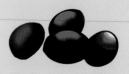

When a Sicilian baby is given its first bath, a few drops of olive oil are added to the water so that the baby will always have a beautiful soft skin.

Native to the Middle East and North Africa, olives produce an oil known for its purity. Offering the olive branch was a symbol of peace and goodwill, and for the same reason winners in the Olympic Games in ancient Greece were crowned with olive branches.

The *savon baladi* of the Middle East and North Africa, used as both soap and shampoo, consists of the residue left over after making olive oil. This pulp has the consistency of thick, dark honey and is left to harden before being cut into blocks.

A Weekly Hair Conditioner

Work warm olive oil through the hair and scalp. Cover your head with a plastic cap and a warm towel and leave for a couple of hours or even, if you have staying power, overnight.

A Cure for Dandruff

Work olive oil into the scalp, avoiding the hair; leave it on for half an hour or so and shampoo it out.

A Persian Face Mask

Mix 1 tablespoon of olive oil with an egg yolk. Apply to the face, leave on for 20 minutes and rinse off with lukewarm water.

An Olive and Honey Treatment for the Hands and Nails

Soak your hands in a bowl of warm water and scrub the nails clean. After drying, dip the nails in warm olive or almond oil for 5 minutes; then massage the oil into the hands, paying attention to the backs and fingers. A teaspoonful of honey can be added to the oil to make a richer treatment. Wrap your hands in a warm towel for 5 minutes, remove and massage your hands once again with oil. If you're doing this in the evening, you may like to put on a pair of cotton gloves and keep the mixture on all night.

FOOD FOR THE FACE

Looking back on her life in Beirut forty years ago, a Lebanese friend told me: 'I remember an old woman I used to know. Whenever she was cooking, whenever she was cutting up fruit or vegetables, she used to dab a little bit on her face! So when she was cutting up a cucumber or a potato, she would rub some of the juice on her skin. She also used strawberries, bananas, even yoghurt. This woman has the most beautiful soft skin I've ever seen, even today when she's very old. Recently I took her a box of natural beauty products I'd bought here in London, and I can tell you, she really looked down her nose at them!'

Any nutritious food which benefits the body when eaten is likely to have a similar effect when applied externally to the skin. Some food, however (like onions, which are reputedly wonderful for banishing wrinkles), are unlikely contenders for use as a cosmetic.

'I remember my great-great-grandmother,' my Lebanese friend went on. 'She used to collect eggshells. She would wash and dry them, then make them into a powder and add water. She used this paste as a cleanser and moisturizer, and also to lighten her skin.'

When she was young, my friend used a face cleanser made of natural clay found in the mountains of Lebanon. Once, when she had injured her knee, she discovered another use for this clay. The wound was swollen, and after she had unsuccessfully tried several modern products prescribed by her doctor, a friend suggested that she use the clay instead. 'I collected it and left it outside for a couple of days to dry and absorb the rays of the sun. Then I made up a paste and left it in the sun again for a couple of hours. I spread it all over my knee, put my feet up and sat there for a few hours. Well, you may not believe this, but when I washed it off my knee was completely dry! The clay had soaked up all the humidity!'

Indian women use buttermilk and goat's milk to cleanse and nourish the face. Another Indian remedy is *gram* (chick-pea flour mixed with water or oil). One woman I spoke to, whose mother has used *gram* all her life, commented: 'When I go out with her, people often think she's my sister, her skin is so soft and smooth!'

In many Middle Eastern countries yoghurt is used as a face mask base, especially for those with dry skin. In fact, if you have olive oil, lemons, yoghurt, eggs, fruit, honey and oatmeal in your larder you have all the ingredients you need for a soft, well-nourished skin, without having to resort to expensive commercial products.

Fruit and vegetables contain an abundance of trace elements, enzymes and vitamins. They are the most nutritious and restorative of all foods, and many dieticians are of the opinion that the best diet is one consisting largely of raw plant food and juices.

Applied externally to the skin, raw fruit and vegetables have varying effects, sometimes acid, sometimes alkaline. Our skin is protected by an acid mantle which wards off infection and if we are healthy our skin will naturally produce its own acid mantle within a few hours of washing. But the passage of time, swimming and too much washing all tend to destroy this mantle.

Fruit Moisturizers

Fresh fruit and vegetable juice patted directly onto the face serves as an instant moisturizer.

Fruits which have the most neutral effect: cucumber, watermelon, fig and banana.

Fruits for dry skin: cantaloup and honeydew melon, olive, lettuce and carrot.

Fruits which help boost acidity: lime, lemon, grape, strawberry, pineapple, grapefruit and apple.

Squeeze or pat these foods onto the face, allow them to dry and wash them off with tepid water. Or mix 2 tablespoons of any of these fruits with a neutral blender such as honey.

Face Masks

Face masks are best left on for 20 to 30 minutes. Relax with your feet up on cushions so that they are higher than your head and place a slice of cucumber over each eyelid.

For an oily skin use buttermilk, yoghurt, whipped egg white, clays and earths.

For a dry skin use banana, sour cream or egg yolk mixed with 5 or 6 drops of cider vinegar or a dollop of oil. Oatmeal mixed with the juice of a grapefruit is another effective face mask.

A RICH AVOCADO FACE MASK. Pulp half the fruit and add 4 dessertspoons of almond oil together with the contents of a vitamin E capsule. Add 6 dessertspoons of double cream. Apply to the face, avoiding the area around the eyes. Leave on for 10 to 15 minutes. Rinse off with warm water.

A TUNISIAN MELON FACE MASK. Scoop out the centre of a honeydew melon (the pips and stringy pith) and mash it up in a pestle and mortar. Apply to the face and leave to dry, then rinse off.

A PERSIAN STRAWBERRY FACE PACK. Here is the most delicious of all face masks, an old remedy which is also said to banish wrinkles. Crush fresh strawberries and mix them with beaten egg whites and rosewater. Apply to the face and leave to dry; then rinse off with a parsley or watercress wash. This is a wonderfully fragrant face pack and will leave the skin with a rosy glow.

CUCUMBER REMEDIES. Slices of peeled cucumber placed on the eyelids help soothe and rest the eyes. There is a hormone in cucumber which makes it an anti-wrinkle aid, and this humble vegetable also has good pore-closing and cleansing properties. It can be lathered on the face after a facial steam bath, or used before steaming the face as a light cleanser.

For a toner, mash a whole peeled cucumber. Add 1 teaspoon of witch-hazel, 1 teaspoon of rosewater and the beaten frothy white of an egg. Keep this in the fridge. You can also add ¼ teaspoon of honey, which is antiseptic and will help nourish and cleanse the skin, and the same quantity of yoghurt.

Flower Water Astringents

After using a face pack, the pores of the skin can be closed with an astringent floral water such as rosewater, or a combination of rosewater and lemon juice or orange flower water.

You can buy inexpensive bottles of flower water in groceries selling Middle Eastern foods and cosmetics. It is used not only as a cleanser but for fainting and nausea and as a flavouring in food and drink.

You can make your own flower water by using 50 ml (170 fl. oz) of bottled spring water to which 10 drops of essential oil (either a single fragrance or in combination) have been added. For a dry skin use geranium and lavender; for an oily skin use bergamot and lavender.

REMEDIES FOR MINOR AILMENTS

Burns

The aloe vera cactus, which grows wild in East and South Africa and the West Indies, has thick leaves which can be sliced diagonally across in thin strips. Between each slice you will find a glutinous gel, and when these strips are laid on sunburnt skin and wounds they will help soothe and heal it.

Mosquito Deterrent

In the Caribbean, women rub the juice of fresh limes all over the body to keep mosquitoes at bay.

Sore Throat

Slice an onion and cover it with honey. Leave this mixture to soak overnight and it will produce a thin liquid which you can drink when you wake up in the morning. It is an excellent cure for sore throats.

Congested Nose

The Indian yogic practice of neti *is a procedure designed to cleanse the body of toxins and promote good health. Neti is a kind of douche which cleanses the nasal membranes. It is simple to carry out, and very effective in relieving a congested nose and helping you breathe freely.*

Fill a small bowl with tepid water and add 1 teaspoon of salt. Pour a little of this solution into your palm and with the other hand block one nostril with your finger. Draw the solution up into the open nostril by making little pumping movements with the back of your throat. The water should go all the way up the nostril and down into the throat until you can taste the salt at the back of your mouth. Now expel the water (together with the debris it has collected) and do the same with the other nostril. Afterwards give your nose a good blow and you will find that your nostrils are completely clear.

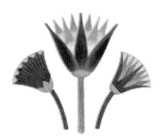

3
Fragrance

By thy scent my soul is ravish'd.
(Sheikh Saadi of Shiraz)

In Egypt there is a little white flower called *full* which pours its fragrance into the air most lavishly at night. The scent of honeysuckle, banana, pineapple and sweet almond, as well as other indefinable fragrances, all seem to be present in this insignificant-looking white flower. In the morning *full* are sold in the market-place to men and women who put them behind their ear or in their hair. The Egyptian expression for 'Good morning', *Sabah al-full*, literally means: 'May your day smell as sweet as this flower.'

There are languages in which the word for 'kiss' is the same as that for 'smell'. Our ritual of kissing or touching opposite cheeks in greeting (in some countries it's once on each cheek and once for luck) is only a way of holding out our face to be sniffed. After all, we aren't so very different from animals who check for danger by sniffing each other on their first encounter. There is a tribe in New Guinea who say goodbye by putting a hand in each other's armpit, then stroking their arm all over themselves, so that they become coated with their friend's scent.

More elusive even than our sense of hearing, smell has an enormous power to awaken our subconscious and stimulate pleasurable thoughts and moods. The limbic system, which recognizes smell, was the first part of our brain to evolve; and though it is the most primitive, it is also in some ways the most sophisticated part of our brain. Scent receptors are the only nerve cells in the brain which repair and renew themselves, but we have very few of them compared to animals, for whom smell is the most acutely developed of the senses. A rabbit can pick up

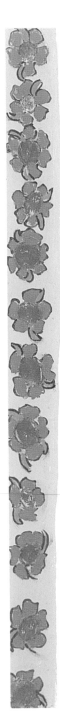

smells through every part of its body and a male silkworm can detect the scent of a female 8 km (5 miles) away. But we humans have only a tiny area with which to pick up scent, hardly more than a few centimetres in size, located in our nose.

Smell is the keenest and most subtle of all our senses, the last to be lost when we die and the one which most eludes definition. Who among us, in an unfamiliar setting, has not had the sudden shock of recognizing, for the first time in years, a smell which brings with it a flood of memories? And who has not had the experience of being violently attracted to someone (or even repelled by them) because of their natural smell? For at certain times we each give off an aroma peculiarly our own, which may prove irresistibly attractive to others yet which is so subtle as to be imperceptible to anyone other than the person who is affected by it. And, what's more, that person is probably unconscious of the fact that this scent is responsible for having caused the attraction in the first place.

Doctors often develop an acute sense of smell through their work and rely on their noses to identify particular illnesses. (Plague is said to smell of apples, measles of freshly plucked feathers and typhoid of mice and freshly baked bread.)

In highly urbanized societies the intellect is considered the most important part of the brain and our other sensory systems are significantly undervalued. There are cultures, though, which place the highest value of all on the limbic system. Some link smell with hearing and have a single word to cover both. The Dogon of Mali talk of 'hearing' smells and divide words by aroma, with good words smelling sweet and bad ones rotten. Certain tribes connect smell and hearing, which reminds us of how perfumers link music and smell, describing a fragrance as a blend of 'notes'.

There is a school of thought which suggests that in the womb our senses mingle; that we see touch, hear smells and feel light, in much the same way as people do under the influence of psychedelic drugs. According to this theory, our brain gradually learns to separate the senses simply in order to avoid sensory overload; yet they remain highly interdependent, with one sense often responsible for triggering the others. Our ability to distinguish the entire range of tastes from savoury to sweet relies closely on our sense of smell; indeed, it is the aroma of food which largely enables us to taste it, and if we have a cold our food loses most of its savour.

Sight and hearing work by analysing waves which bounce off our eyes and ears, but scent reacts with chemicals within the body, making it a far more intimate sense. Most of the time we aren't actively aware of our need for fragrance, yet all our extremes of mood, from euphoria and the sexual urge to fear, pain, fury and recoil come from our sense of smell.

There are certain notes in flowers which echo those present in the human body. The heavy aroma of musk, amber and sandalwood are all present in human pheromones; and these particular fragrances were among the earliest, most popular ones to be used for both personal adornment and religious ceremony.

The Victorians believed perfume was so sexually suggestive that they only used light toilet waters directly on their skin. They reserved the more heady aromas for their clothes. In the West we traditionally prefer light, flowery scents and use perfume sparingly, dabbing it behind the ears and on our pulse points. In our surroundings we hardly use it at all. But in Asian and Eastern cultures women may use a different perfume for each part of the body, or anoint the walls of their homes with scent and deck their beds with fragrant greenery.

Heat increases all our perceptions, especially that of smell, and the hotter the climate the more we crave fragrance and want our perfumes strong. Cinnamon, cloves, myrrh and fenugreek all give off a heady aroma, and all are favourites in the East, where aromatics are used with glorious extravagance.

Indian paisley shawls, popular in nineteenth-century Britain, were packed into boxes with layers of patchouli leaves for transportation to Europe. The original reason for this was to keep moths away, but exporters soon realized that they would be unable to sell the shawls if they were not impregnated with this powerful, heavy perfume, which came to be part of their attraction.

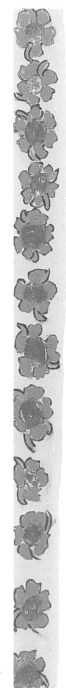

A SHORT HISTORY OF FRAGRANCE

Fragrance masks the smell of decay and death, and it is no accident that ancient Egypt, a culture obsessed with death and immortality, was renowned for its manufacture of fine perfumes. In pharaonic times Egyptians were urged by popular decree to use perfume. Nor, as we may think, was this a luxury for the wealthy or for women only. Perfume expands the wearer's presence and also their territory and men in the ancient world were great enthusiasts of perfume. During the reign of Seti I, scented oils were issued to the army. During the reign of Rameses III, the grave-diggers of Thebes are even reported to have gone on strike in protest against a decline in the amount of perfume supplied to them. At dinner parties Egyptian men were offered their choice of perfumes at the door and given garlands of flowers to hang round their necks. Cretan athletes anointed themselves with particular oils before the games and Homer records the courtesy of offering visitors a bath with aromatic oils. In ancient Rome the wealthy soaked their cloths in perfume and anointed their pets with it, and even gladiators used scented lotions before stepping into the ring for a fight.

Aromatics were used in religious rituals for their emotional and uplifting qualities long before they were used for personal adornment. For thousands of years Indian yogis have taught that incense and perfumed oils should be used to stimulate creativity and help heighten spiritual awareness, and in many other societies too, aromatics have been used as a link between the physical and spiritual worlds.

The ancient Egyptians used scented oils for massage. One of their most famous aromatic formulas, popular also with the Greeks and Romans, was *kyphi*, a concoction of sixteen herbs and wood resins. It is thought that these included cassia, cyprus, calamus, myrrh, mastic, spikenard, henna, cinnamon, juniper, terebinth and raisins. Saffron and frankincense are two other possible additions. These ingredients were pounded and sifted together, steeped in wine, then beaten to a pulp and left to thicken. This paste was mixed with honey and stored in earthenware jars. The Romans were the most lavish of all in their love of perfume. They applied a different scent to every part of the body, and at banquets they used to anoint the feet of guests with scented oils.

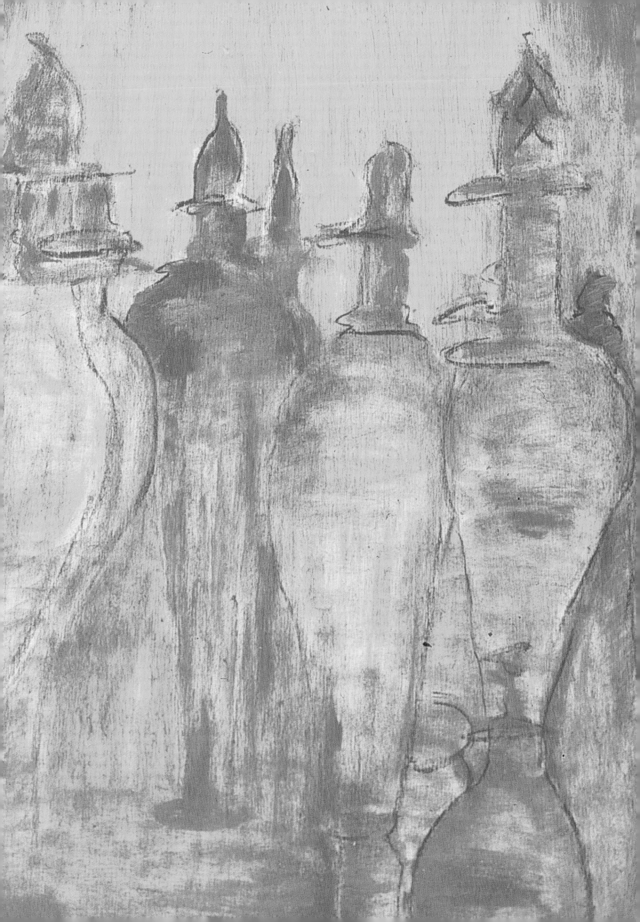

Spices and aromatics were a crucial commodity and a staple of trade, and were almost as valuable as gold and silver. Indeed, the control of the spice trade, with its related taxes and tariffs, resulted in the rise to power of successive countries at different epochs. Egypt was one country which owed its ascendancy to this trade. It was superseded by Greece and Rome and then, from the seventh century onwards, by Arab-Islamic countries. They took control of areas producing the raw materials for aromatics as well as the secret trade routes which led to them through India, Ethiopia and Somalia. There were ports situated all along the coast of the Red Sea supplying trade vessels with this priceless commodity, and nearly every day spice-laden caravans made their way up and down the coastline, always susceptible to attacks by marauding tribes for their valuable cargo.

The way perfumes were made and used in the ancient world was recorded in Egyptian manuscripts and on the bas-reliefs of tombs. Roots were crushed to give up their aromatic qualities, but extracting the fragrance of flowers, leaves and woods was a more complicated business. First they were steeped in oil and water; then the resulting essence was skimmed off and combined with a base oil such as olive, almond or sesame. Ointment, on the other hand, was made by placing a plant in oil or fat and leaving it out in the sun for a few days, during which time the carrier substance became infused with the fragrance of the plant.

It was not until the eleventh century that the process of distillation was discovered, making it possible to create strong, long-lasting perfumes without the use of a heavy base oil. Distillation is credited to the eleventh-century Persian physician and philosopher Avicenna (Ibn Sina) and was later refined by the Arabs, who also discovered how to make alcohol. Knights fighting in the Crusades brought back essential oils from the Middle East, and the popularity of these oils led to the manufacture of perfume in Europe in the twelfth century. Even without the benefit of distillation, perfumes made in ancient Egypt have proved wonderfully enduring. In 1922, when the tomb of Tutankhamun was opened, archeologists found some containers of ointment. As the lids were removed for the first time in thousands of years, a long pent-up whisper of delicate fragrance was released.

Our ancestors believed that flowers contained a divine spirit. As smoke rose to heaven, they reasoned, so the perfumed smoke of incense could carry their prayers to the gods. Their prayers would be all the more welcome in that, not only would they smell sweet, but the gods could nourish themselves on the smoke. Our very word 'perfume' (from the Latin *per fumum*, 'through smoke') reflects this original belief.

In Babylon many thousands of years ago the idea originated of mixing perfumed oils with mortar for buildings, so that in the heat of the day a delicate fragrance would emanate from the walls. For religious processions in Constantinople (present-day Istanbul) the streets were washed and decked with fragrant bunches of myrtle, rosemary, ivy and box. Incense burners were placed in the doors and windows of houses all along the route and sweet perfumes were sprinkled over dignitaries as they passed by. *Kyphi* was used for religious purposes and burned in the home at night for its somnolent effect, as well as to induce dreams. Its possible narcotic qualities would have derived from the inclusion of calamus, a toxic, highly sedative substance which can cause hallucinations.

Musk

She captures your heart with the flash of her smile,
Her mouth sweet to the kiss, sweet to the taste,
Like a draft of musk from a spiceman's pouch.
('Antarah, *al-Mu'allaqat*)

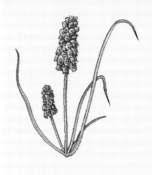

In the ancient world, musk was mixed in with the mortar that went into the building of palaces and mosques (on one occasion 1,000 sackfuls went into a single minaret). The mosque of Kara Ahmet Pasha in Istanbul is known as 'Iparie', meaning musk, because so great a quantity of this precious fragrance was used in its construction that, to this day, when the sun is at its height, its walls continue to release this scent into the air.

Musk is an endurable fragrance and is used in perfume both as a fixative and to give depth to the lighter floral ingredients.

According to the Qur'an, the water of the gardens of paradise is perfumed with musk and will quench the thirst forever. Musk is to be found in such abundance in paradise that a houri only has to spit on the ground and the place where she has spat will straightaway be turned into musk. The principal delight of the Islamic paradise is the presence of nymphs and houris who are partly made out of this sweet, heavy scent; these female sprites are the chief reward of men who enter paradise. (The Qur'an does not tell us what will be women's reward when they enter the afterlife.)

Musk is said to stimulate the libido and the Victorians thought it reeked of debauchery. Real musk has a male smell and is obtained from the penile shaft of a small deer. Although it can be extracted without hurting the deer, the animal is usually killed to obtain it. Today synthetic musk is now widely used in its place. Musky smells are similar to those used in incense to invoke religious rapture.

Napoleon was so enamoured of the Empress Josephine's natural smell that he once wrote to her: 'I'll be home in three days. Don't wash.' But unfortunately Josephine had a passion for the smell of musk. Even the wallpaper in her bedroom was doused with this heavy aroma. Filling the room with musk to welcome Napoleon home from the wars and put him in an amorous mood, she unfortunately ended up by giving him a splitting headache instead. (We are told that Napoleon ordered the walls to be doused with lime to get rid of the scent.)

To Create a Perfumed Oil
Fill a glass bottle with herbs or flowers, top it up with a light, fragrance-free oil and stopper it. Leave it in a warm place for a few weeks.

ESSENTIAL OILS

One of the most enjoyable discoveries I've made in the past few years is the existence of essential oils. They can be used in the bath, in massage, to help you sleep if your mind is racing and to perfume rooms. When I'm writing, if I don't want to stimulate my brain with endless cups of coffee I burn a couple of drops of basil oil in a fragrancer on my desk. This creates a sharp, fresh smell which keeps my brain awake without the knock-out effect of too much coffee. Sometimes I give essential oils as gifts and it's very gratifying when a friend calls up and says: 'Those oils are the best present you've ever given me!'

One of the ways essential oils work, especially in massage or in the bath, is that they are slowly absorbed by the skin and taken into the bloodstream. The properties of different aromatics take varying lengths of time to be released after they have been applied directly to the body, and modern medicine has lately begun to look seriously at their possible benefits. Experiments have shown that the typhoid bacillus can be killed in twelve minutes with cinnamon oil, in twenty-five minutes with clove oil and in under an hour with geranium.

The use of fragrance to heal the body is part of an ancient wisdom which we are in the process of rediscovering today. Essential oils can stimulate our energy and bolster our confidence, and research has demonstrated their effectiveness as an aid to relaxation and to reduce blood pressure and stress.

A French psychologist working with patients who found it hard to recall long-suppressed memories found that when they inhaled the smell from cotton-wool balls soaked in specific essential oils, long-buried memories resurfaced. Using these oils as an alternative to prescription drugs for particular ailments has proved effective and has the obvious advantage of not having any of the side-effects connected with allopathic drugs; for the latter have a gradually deadening effect on the body's immune system, as well as being known for wearing away its ability to respond to sensation.

Unlike synthetic drugs, essential oils do not target specific bodily organs and become stored in them. Instead it is thought that the organs themselves attract and absorb these oils, as they do other nutrients. It seems that particular parts of the body draw specific oils to them; thus sandalwood appears to lodge in (and hence have a strong effect on) the bladder, while neroli and ylang-ylang have a greater effect on the nervous system.

For babies who have suffered violence and neglect and have been removed from their natural parents, it has been found that, when all attempts to help them thrive have failed, the only therapy they will respond to is massage with essential oils.

Some oils have a relaxing, sedating, even aphrodisiac effect; others are stimulating and energizing. When used in particular combinations they may bring out each other's properties more strongly than when they are used alone.

How to Use Essential Oils

Essential oils are seventy times more concentrated than their original plant form, so a very small amount of them is needed. With essential oils it isn't true that the more you use the better the results will be; in fact the reverse may be the case. There are also a few oils which are toxic and which may make your skin itch. If you are at all sensitive to a particular oil, simply stop using it.

It is worth using genuine essential oils, even though you can buy the cheaper, synthetic variety. Synthetic oils may be less costly but they are never the same as those which come from natural herbs and flowers. This is because scientists are only able to analyse and identify certain components of a fragrance. There are always elements in the spectrum which elude them, and it is the action of the entire spectrum working together which creates the unique effect of a particular oil.

Some products masquerade as pure essential oils when they are diluted with base oils such as almond or grapeseed. It is easy to tell if an essential oil has been adulterated in this way by comparing a few drops on a piece of blotting paper, side by side with some drops of a pure essential oil: the base oils will sit in an oily patch, while the pure essential oils will impregnate the blotting paper and then evaporate, without leaving any oily stain behind.

In the Bath

Disperse 10 drops of essential oil in the water. The oil takes effect as it becomes absorbed by the skin into the bloodstream.

   Some relaxing oils: lavender, bergamot, sandalwood.
   Some stimulating oils: rosewood, orange, geranium.

Home-made Perfume and Cologne

About ninety per cent of the price of a bottle of perfume goes towards packaging, promotion, profits and other costs. Only a tiny ten per cent of the money we pay is spent on the raw ingredients which make up the fragrance. Today, more and more perfumes are made from laboratory-produced chemicals rather than natural oils. This has resulted in an ever-increasing number of new products, a bewildering array of loudly trumpeted perfumes, many of which, to my own nose, have an unmistakable whiff of lavatory cleaner about them.

While many commercial perfumes result from the subtle blending of a hundred or more fragrances, some of the most popular ones include no more than three or four. Although it isn't really possible to devise a sophisticated perfume in the home, we can certainly make a simple one for ourselves, using a few of our favourite essential oils, with the bonus of knowing that we are applying natural rather than synthetic smells to our body. Indeed, several of my Middle Eastern and Indian friends wear just one fragrance, rose and jasmine being the most popular.

Pure alcohol is the usual medium for making perfume and cologne, but is not available to the general public. Instead you can use the relatively odourless vodka or, if you do not care for the alcoholic smell, you can make up a perfume using a jojoba base. (Vegetable oils are not a good medium for making perfume, as they tend to go off; jojoba, on the other hand, is a liquid wax and hence does not oxidize.)

Use 20 drops essential oils to 10 ml (35 fl. oz) jojoba oil.

Or use a ratio of 15 to 30 per cent essential oils to 70 per cent alcohol/water.

You can also make perfume and eau de cologne using essential oils together with distilled water (which you can buy from the chemist), spring or bottled water, or using a combination of spring water and vodka. The ratio is 30 ml (100 fl. oz) water to 70 ml (240 fl. oz) of 100 per cent vodka .

Use a sterilized bottle, preferably made of dark glass, which causes less evaporation than clear.

Add the essential oils to the vodka, stirring to disperse them, and leave to stand for a couple of days. Then add the water, shaking the bottle to mix the ingredients well, and leave, preferably for a few weeks, before using.

Fragrances: scent is so much to do with individual preference that I think it is more fun to experiment than to make up a recommended formula, but there are certain essential oils which are commonly used in perfume-making.

For a heady scent, rose mingles well with geranium, rosewood and sandalwood.

For a lighter scent, a combination of bergamot, lemon, rosewood and orange go well together.

Vanilla, benzoin and lavender provide a good link between floral and citrus essences.

If you are using the most expensive oils, such as rose or jasmine, you need only 2 to 4 drops.

Other oils used in popular commercial brands of perfume include: ylang-ylang, vetiver, carnation. cinnamon, ginger, neroli, frankincense, orris root, mandarin and tuberose.

Perfumed Oils for Massage

Add a total of 24 drops of essential oil to 50 ml (170 fl. oz) of a carrier oil. The best carrier oils are light, odourless and clear. For this reason olive oil, even though it has many beneficial properties, isn't best suited as a carrier oil; its heavy fragrance will overpower any perfume you want to add to it. Ideal carrier oils are sweet almond, apricot kernel, grapeseed, sunflower and avocado. Calendula oil, which is Egyptian in origin and comes from marigold, is excellent but expensive. In India they favour mustard seed oil.

Baby oil is unsuitable for massage. It is a mineral – as opposed to vegetable – oil and has low powers of penetration. Instead of becoming absorbed into the body it will sit on the surface of the skin in a light film.

Make up your own mixture, using essential oils to suit the type of massage you want to give, whether relaxing or stimulating.

A relaxing massage oil:
   15 drops sandalwood
   5 drops ylang-ylang
   5 drops geranium or lavender
   50 ml (170 fl. oz) carrier oil.

A massage oil to relieve stress:
   10 drops clary sage
   10 drops lemon
   5 drops marjoram
   50 ml (170 fl. oz) carrier oil.

A rejuvenating massage oil:
   6 drops juniper
   12 drops lavender
   7 drops rosemary
   50 ml (170 fl. oz) carrier oil.

For the Face
A moisturizer:
   12 drops rosewood
   10 drops bergamot
   2 drops juniper or ylang-ylang
   50 ml (170 fl. oz) carrier oil.

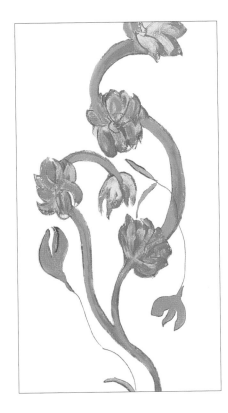

A night oil:
  8 drops sandalwood
  10 drops lavender
  4 drops ylang-ylang
  2 drops geranium
  50 ml (170 fl. oz) carrier oil.

A facial sauna:
sprinkle 2 to 3 drops of essential oil in a
bowl of boiled water:
    for dull skin use lavender or rosemary
    for an oily skin use geranium
    for a mature skin use rose.

When I'm travelling, I take with me
laven-der, tea-tree and rosemary as remedies for basic ailments, together with
rose for its intoxicating fragrance.

Lavender

Lavender is the most versatile essential oil and the only one which many
aromatherapists advise using neat on the skin, where it is especially effective against
burns and scalds. Because all essential oils are concentrated, only a few drops are
needed at a time – using too many will not make the treatment more effective.

Lavender has antibiotic and antiseptic qualities, and if you are feeling frazzled
and tense, a few drops in the bath before going to bed has a wonderfully relaxing
effect, both on the muscles and the mind. Using lavender oil in the bath also helps
build up the immune system and contributes to the healing process when you have
flu or are under the weather. It can be applied neat against sunburn, mosquito bites,
fish bites, plant stings and swollen areas of the body. It is said to neutralize the sting
of the black widow spider if 10 drops are applied to the affected area every 10 minutes
before reaching hospital.

If I could only take one oil with me to my desert island, without question it would be lavender.

Tea-tree

Tea-tree has miraculous antiseptic qualities and has become the subject of considerable research. Its anti-bacterial, anti-viral and anti-fungal properties make it effective in many medical conditions, including toothache, candida, sunburn, colds, catarrh, cuts and wounds.

Rosemary

After a strenuous dance session, I find that soaking in a bath with some rosemary and lavender oil is excellent for my tired muscles. Rosemary is a stimulant and can be used for muscular sprains, arthritis, rheumatism, depression, coughs, flu and headaches, among other conditions. A rosemary rinse is also a popular old-fashioned hair care remedy for dark hair.

SOME ESSENTIAL OILS AND THEIR THERAPEUTIC USES

Antiseptic/Disinfectant

lavender, pine, thyme, bergamot, eucalyptus, juniper, geranium.

Boosting the Immune System

lavender, geranium, tea-tree.

Fighting Infection

eucalyptus, lavender, tea-tree, lemon, clove, thyme.

Stimulant and Aid to Concentration

basil, bergamot, juniper, cardamom.

Calming Stress and Anxiety and for Relaxing

lavender, neroli, camomile, mint (for stomach), rose, vetiver, juniper.

Sedative

neroli, lavender, marjoram.

Clearing Bacteria and Viruses from the Air

bergamot, tea-tree, cypress, lavender, rosemary, oregano.

Insomnia

An old Persian remedy recommends sprinkling a few drops of lavender or marjoram oil on the pillow or in the bath. Both oils are effective, though lavender has a generally soothing scent and marjoram is a more powerful soporific.

Colds and Flu

Tea-tree, eucalyptus and lemon, inhaled in the bath or over a basin of hot water (cover your head with a towel).

To clear your nose, place a drop of rosemary or eucalyptus on a handkerchief and inhale whenever you can.

Or make up a massage oil using a total of 6 drops, combining lemon, eucalyptus and rosemary, and dilute in a teaspoon of carrier oil. This can be massaged all over the sinus area, neck, upper back and chest. Another combination of oils used in this way is eucalyptus, lavender and bergamot.

Alternatively, take a bath using the above oils.

Bleeding Gums

Dilute 2 drops of lemon and eucalyptus and 1 drop of lavender in 1 teaspoon of brandy. Add it to a glass of warm water and use it as a mouthwash. DO NOT SWALLOW.

Burns

Bathe the affected area in ice-cold water for 10 minutes. Then apply 2 drops of neat lavender oil directly to the skin. Make a cold compress by soaking a clean piece of gauze or material in cold water. Add 5 drops of lavender oil to this compress and cover the burnt area with it. If you do not have anything handy to make a compress, simply apply a few drops of neat oil at regular intervals.

Cuts and Wounds

Bathe with warm water containing 5 drops lavender and 2 drops tea-tree. Put 3 drops lavender onto a strip of gauze and cover the cut with it. Renew twice daily, and after the third day expose the skin to the air, if the wound is sufficiently healed.

Mouth Ulcers

Make up a mouthwash using a glass of warm water to which you have added 1 teaspoon of the following combination: 2 drops peppermint, 4 drops lemon, 2 drops geranium and 2 drops thyme diluted in 1 dessertspoon of brandy. Rinse the mouth thoroughly but DO NOT SWALLOW.

Or put 1 drop myrrh onto a cotton bud and apply to the ulcer several times a day.

Sore Throat

Mix 3 drops lavender, 1 drop thyme and 2 drops camomile in a bowl of hot water and use as a steam inhalation. Or you can massage the neck and behind the ears with 1 drop thyme, 2 drops lemon and 5 drops camomile mixed with 1 teaspoon of carrier oil.

Toothache

Add 1 drop clove oil to a cotton bud and apply it to the gums around the troublesome tooth.

Hangover

Drink a cup of warm water and honey in which 2 drops of fennel have been diluted.

Insect Repellent

Citronella oil is especially useful in warding off insects. Rosemary and eucalyptus are also said to be effective.

Flying and Jet Lag

To guard against jet lag, before leaving home have a bath with a couple of drops of peppermint or eucalyptus; or else use these same oils on a flannel and wipe it all over your body after taking a shower.

For the journey: if you're nervous of flying, take a handkerchief sprinkled with a drop of lavender, camomile or geranium. When you feel anxious take a sniff, then lie back, close your eyes and relax.

On arrival at your destination and before going to bed, take a bath in which you've floated a few drops of lavender oil. Or else massage your face, neck and upper back with a palmful of carrier oil containing a few drops of lavender. It's good, too, to massage some of this oil over other parts of your body that may have stiffened up during the journey.

Thrush

Taking a bath in essential oils can help clear thrush. Use a combination of 1 drop savory, 2 drops lavender and 2 drops patchouli in the bath water.

Diarrhoea

The main problem which comes with diarrhoea is the possibility of dehydration and the consequent loss of salt and sugar to the body. Combine 1 l (2 pt) of bottled water with 8 drops of lemon essential oil, ½ teaspoon of salt and 8 teaspoons of sugar. Drink a glass of this mixture after visits to the toilet.

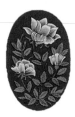

4
Massage

What is the most agreeable of sounds?
The voice of the loved one.
(The *Kama Sutra*)

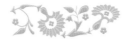

In the opening warm-up to a long dance workshop, I sometimes include a five-minute back massage. Everyone finds a partner of about the same height. One woman stands with her eyes closed while her partner moves one hand slowly but firmly up and down her spine, neck and back. Many of the women at these workshops have never met before and the effect of this silent, meditative few minutes before the hard work of the day begins always has the effect of drawing people closer together and making them feel part of the group. Afterwards there are sighs of contentment. And there is a lot of laughter, because nobody expects to start a day's dancing with something purely pleasurable and relaxing!

Massage as a healing technique is thousands of years old. Murals in a physician's tomb at Saqqara (Egypt), dating back to 2330 BC, suggest that a form of reflexology (pressure-point therapy concentrated on the feet) may have been practised in pharaonic times nearly 2,000 years before Christ.

A form of aromatherapy (massage using infused oils) was practised 5,000 years ago in the ancient world. It played a vital role in the Ayurvedic medical system of India and was part of therapeutic practice in the Middle East for around 4,000 years before it went into decline. In the fifth century BC Hippocrates wrote: 'The physician must be experienced in many things, but assuredly in rubbing . . . For rubbing can bind a joint that is loose and loosen a joint that is too rigid.' The ancient Greeks went to the gymnasium daily and followed up with a massage.

After the fall of the Roman empire it was the Arabs and Persians who

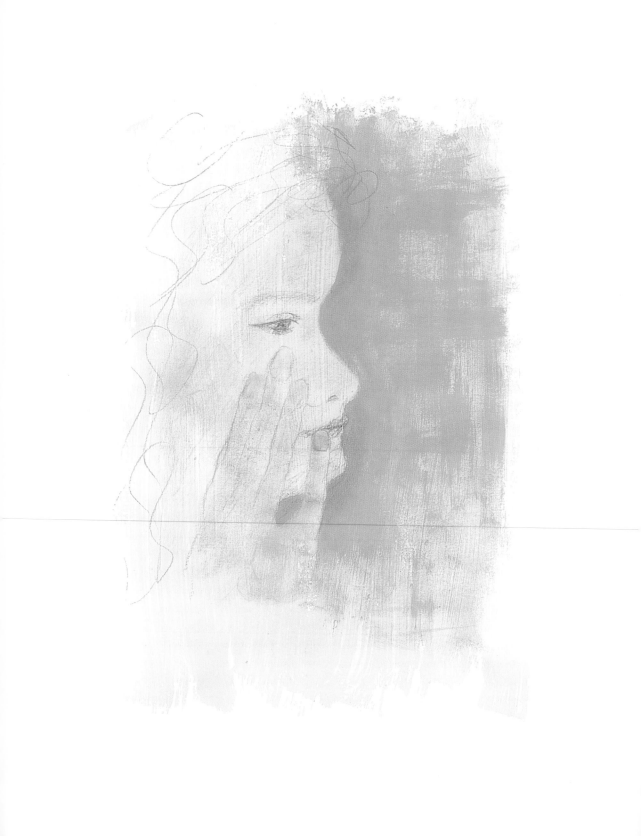

continued to develop the teachings of the classical world. Avicenna wrote that the object of massage was 'to disperse the effete matter found in the muscles and not expelled by exercise'.

Among other forms of massage are shiatsu, which is traditional to Japan, and reflexology. Reflexology was used in Asia for many centuries to diagnose and treat health problems throughout the entire body.

Christianity has always frowned on what is considered indulgence of the flesh and, until recently, massage was considered a purely sexual activity. Helping soothe stress in our friends and family with this form of 'laying on of hands' is still uncommon, but a therapeutic tradition is now becoming established in the Western world. The recent growth of holistic massage and the revival of aromatherapy in the West dates back to the 1960s, when there was an explosion of interest in every aspect of Eastern culture.

BABY MASSAGE

A few years ago I read an article about premature babies written by a male research scientist. He had discovered that if the babies were massaged for fifteen minutes in their incubators three times a day they gained weight forty-five per cent faster than babies who were left alone – not because they ate more, but because the sense of touch had such a beneficial effect on their metabolism. The findings of another experiment revealed that the nervous systems of premature babies who were massaged developed more rapidly, enabling them to be discharged from hospital earlier.

To many of us it may seem glaringly obvious that touch soothes and promotes well-being; that leaving a newborn baby alone for long periods at a time, whether or not it is premature, can only produce anxiety rather than encourage it to thrive.

In the womb a baby floats in warm water and is continually rocked by its mother's movement. Stripped of this reassuring movement at birth, put in a separate room to sleep, left alone for hours, it is no wonder that babies cry out in fear when they wake up in the night, alone in the dark and with no reassuring presence beside them.

Among the Wolof of Senegal, a visitor is immediately given a baby to hold, sometimes before anyone says a word. In this way the baby becomes the natural intermediary between people. Friends of mine who have travelled with their babies, particularly women travelling alone in the developing world, comment on how easy it is to make contact with strangers, who are instinctively drawn towards babies.

Among the Bornu of Nigeria, when a woman gives birth all her birth helpers heat their hands over hot coals and each in turn holds and strokes the new baby.

In Morocco in the first week after birth a baby is never left alone, for fear an evil spirit will take it away and substitute one of its own offspring. Every day the mother is massaged with henna, walnut bark and kohl to help her recover. The baby is also massaged with different lotions using alum, marjoram, mastic, mint, water and oil. If it cries, it is held in the soothing smoke of incense.

In India, Africa and other tropical zones many women carry their babies around constantly with them, and baby massage, with its soothing skin-to-skin contact, is an integral part of mothering. Oiling protects the skin, while stroking and gently stretching the body are believed to help the baby grow stronger and keep it supple.

General Hints for Baby Massage

A good time to give a baby a massage is after a bath, when the baby is still warm. Make sure that the room too is very warm.

Give your hands and fingers a stretch before you begin and rub them together to heat them up. Leave your legs bare so that the baby has extra skin contact with you.

You can work comfortably on the floor with your legs outstretched and the baby lying face up in your lap with its feet pointing towards you. It will be more relaxed if it can see your face, and from its expression you will be able to tell whether it is enjoying what you are doing! It's a good idea to lay a large towel underneath you both, in case the baby relaxes its bottom muscles in more ways than you would like!

Keep your movements rhythmic and flowing and above all gentle. The penetrating, deep tissue massage which we like as adults is designed to unlock deeply held muscle tension. A baby is so much more sensitive and delicate, and in any case, hopefully doesn't yet have need of such rigorous treatment! Massaging a baby is designed more to reassure than to get rid of knots.

Finally, keep the massage short – 10 to 20 minutes is enough.

Indian Baby Massage

Heat a light vegetable oil such as almond or coconut by placing it in a pan of hot water.

Slowly rub a little oil all over the front of the baby, leaving out the face. Mould your hand to the baby's soft little contours as you spread the oil.

Stroke it gently all over in a soothing way, from top to toe.

When massaging the arms and legs, complete one limb before moving on to another. Take hold of one of the baby's hands and squeeze its arm gently from shoulder to wrist with your other hand. After repeating this on the other side you may like to squeeze both arms simultaneously, one with each hand, all the way down the body.

You can use a similar technique on the legs, this time taking hold of one of the baby's feet with one of your hands and squeezing gently down from the thigh with the other.

Now you can rub the baby's tummy, with soft strokes, alternating one hand after the other, drawing each hand towards you. Then stroke around the belly button with feather-light strokes in a clockwise direction. Take care around the umbilical cord.

Turn the baby over on its tummy and either lie it across your legs or lean back in a chair with the baby resting on your chest.

Stroke up and down the back, soothing the baby's spinal nerves, and finish off with long strokes starting at the top. Now gently squeeze its bottom.

GIVING AND RECEIVING A MASSAGE

Receiving a massage is like entering a secret garden of extrasensory perception. If it's good it can leave us in a state so relaxed and blissful that we become ultra-aware of everything around us; we become aware of sounds that we would

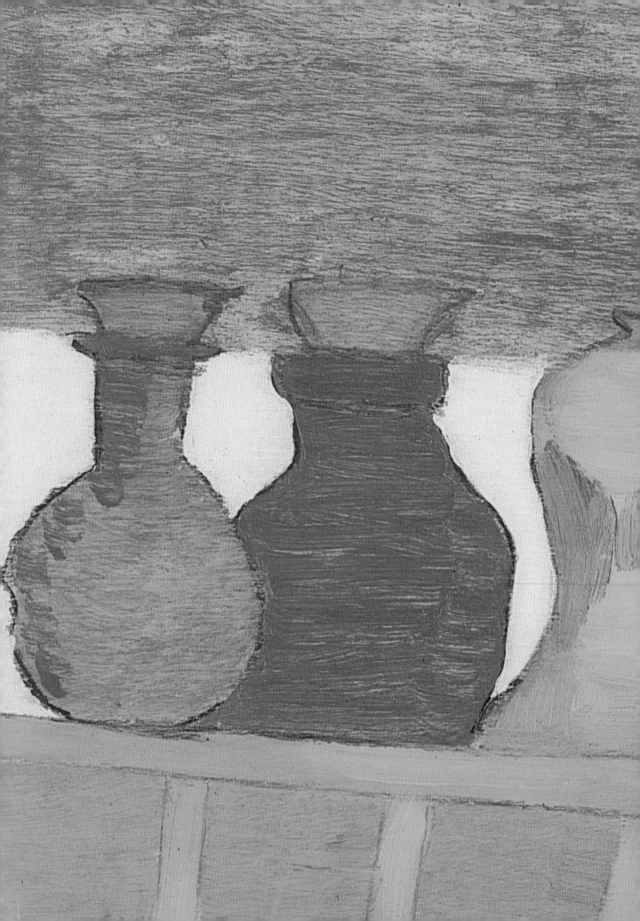

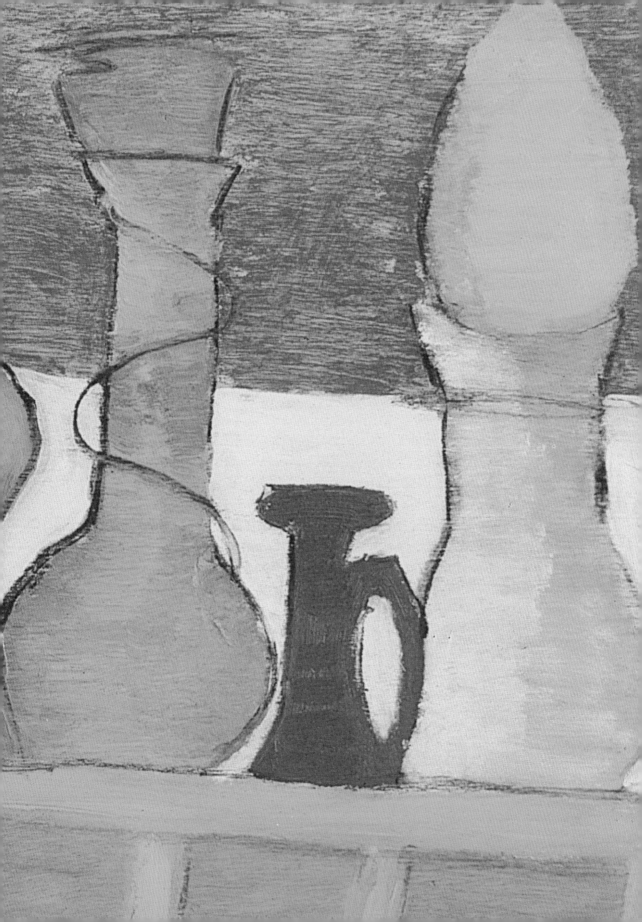

otherwise fail to notice; we breathe more slowly; and when we look in the mirror all the lines on our face seem to have vanished!

Massage is a two-way process which can be as relaxing for the masseur as for the recipient. This is especially so if we are using essential oils, for the masseur too is inhaling the fragrance and absorbing their beneficial qualities. For someone who has never experienced massage, a face, neck or foot massage is a good initiation. Even if you only have fifteen or twenty minutes to spare (perhaps at the end of a session at the steam baths), that's long enough.

The most commonly used technique is known as 'Swedish' massage. This system was developed by a nineteenth-century Swede, Per Henrik Ling, who created a synthesis of the techniques once used in China, Egypt, Greece and Rome.

I have seen many manuals which include a section on self-massage. But in my opinion self-massage is something of a contradiction in terms. For one thing, the beneficial effects of massage come from total relaxation, emptying your mind and giving yourself up to the sensation of touch. If you are trying to massage yourself your brain must necessarily be active, and in this situation you cannot truly relax. Besides which, there are large areas of your own body which you simply won't be able to reach! A major benefit of massage is that it is a form of communication with someone else and (whether you're paying for it or not) all their energies are directed towards your well-being.

In massage there are various types of strokes. Some are intended to be purely relaxing, others invigorating, and still others go more deeply to help dissolve crystalline toxins and relieve muscles which have developed knots of tension. Masseurs who are experienced in detecting these knots and crystals will concentrate on trying to disperse them.

Needless to say, the ideal time to receive a massage is after you've had a bath or shower and when you don't have any energetic activities to rush on to.

You don't have to be an expert to offer someone a massage, but following a few basic rules will make all the difference towards it being enjoyable:

Pressure is highly individual: some people like to feel their muscles are being given a good work-out and they are disturbed by too light a touch; others are so sensitive they can take only the lightest pressure. Never suffer in silence when you are receiving a massage. If you want a deeper or lighter pressure, ask for it rather than expect your masseur or masseuse to read your thoughts!

It's best not to talk when you're giving a massage. This is because you want your partner to focus on your touch, rather than your thoughts. It's hard to relax and abandon ourselves to physical sensation if we feel a verbal response is called for. Your partner may find it easier to empty their mind if soft music is playing, but check first; they may prefer silence. It goes without saying that loud, highly rhythmic music is not conducive to relaxation.

If the oil is cold, warm it up before you begin by standing the bottle in a pan of hot water. Pour a little oil into your hands (which you may also need to warm beforehand) and rub it in before beginning to apply it to your partner's skin. Don't use too much – the object isn't to grease your partner up for the frying pan.

If you are giving a full body massage, make sure the room is warm. Your partner will feel colder than you because they will be lying still; so have a sheet and light blankets to cover them, if need be.

Make sure your partner is lying in a relaxed position, with their body straight, arms resting loosely beside them (some people tend to lie with their legs crooked, so check and straighten them out before you begin). A bed isn't an ideal surface, but will do. A table with some blankets to soften the surface is ideal, as you will be able to move freely around it and will thus have more control over the different strokes.

A good way to begin is to cover your partner's body with a soft sheet which you have just warmed. The sensation of heat on the skin will help them relax and is very comforting. Uncover only that part of the body which you are working on at the time: if you leave an arm uncovered when you have finished working on it, it will soon grow cold and your partner will become uncomfortable. At the end leave the room and allow him or her a few minutes to recover and come back down to earth.

Massage Strokes

There are many different massage strokes, and skilful masseurs tend, with experience, to make up their own. The ones I have suggested below are simply a selection which

I have personally experienced over the years and which have felt wonderful to me!
Once you have familiarized yourself with some of the basic strokes, just follow your
intuition.

A useful tip is to mould your hand to the shape of your partner's body, as if your
hand is made of warm liquid. Begin each stroke in the air, so that by the time your
hand makes contact with their body, it will already be moving fluidly. Stroke the
body slowly and firmly (too light and it will tickle) and think of touching rather
than pressing, with your hands moving in a slow, relaxed dance over the skin, moving
imperceptibly from one part of the body to the next.

EFFLEURAGE is a gliding movement using long, continuous strokes. Aim for a
regular rhythm, using long strokes rather than short, jerky ones, and remember to
keep it slow. Moving your hands too fast will make your partner agitated. You can
use both hands together, or one hand after the other; as you lift the first hand off
your partner's body, the second hand takes its place, each stroke slightly overlapping
to create a sense of continuity.

FEATHERING is a light, downward brushing stroke with the fingertips. It is a good
stroke with which to end a deep leg or back massage; it is also a good stroke to use at
the very end of a massage. Your fingers gradually make less and less contact with
your partner's body, and in this way you can let them know that the massage is
coming to an end.

KNEADING, as the name implies, is a lifting, squeezing and rolling movement like
that used in bread-making. It is good for getting to grips with tight, knotted muscles,
especially in the neck, upper back and legs. Lift and gently squeeze the flesh between
the thumbs and fingers of each hand alternately, rocking smoothly from one to the
other in a continuous motion. Remember not to lift the hand entirely off the body
with each stroke.

WRINGING enables you to go more deeply into tense muscles. Resting your hands
on your partner's body, press deeper with your fingers and thumbs, adding a finishing
twist to each stroke.

The Feet

In ancient Egypt a kiss on the foot was considered as gallant as a kiss on the hand, and if any one part of the body deserves to be pampered it's our feet. The foot is an incredibly delicate, as well as hard-working piece of engineering. It has tens of thousands of nerve endings, the opposite ends of which are located all over the body. There is no muscle, gland or organ in our body which doesn't have a corresponding set of nerves in the foot, so when we massage people's feet we are affecting the rest of their body at the same time.

Reflexology involves the application of pressure to the feet alone. Using the thumbs, this pressure is applied to points on the sole of the foot which correspond to specific bodily organs. An experienced reflexologist can diagnose illness by 'reading' the sensitivity or stiffness of these pressure points.

For a foot massage your partner can sit or lie down in front of you, resting one foot in your lap or on one thigh. You may like to place a cushion or pillow under the foot.

Begin by stroking down the front of the foot from the ankles to the toes.

Now use your knuckles to massage the thick soles of the feet. An exquisite stroke is to mould the knuckle to the shape of the foot as it passes from heel to toe.

Go over the sole in small circles, applying firm pressure with the thumbs. Pay special attention to the hard-working spongy ball of the foot. Finish by taking the foot in both hands, one hand on top, the other underneath, and warming it with your hands for a moment before gently releasing it.

The Face and Head

There is a type of face massage which I have only ever received from a beautician friend of mine. It feels absolutely divine and is unlike any other face massage I have ever experienced. (Technically speaking, I am told that it is a combination of deep effleurage and roll-patting.) The hands pass very, very slowly over the face like warm waves, which make me feel as if every line on my face is being eradicated. This particular technique includes, at one point, the use of individual fingers in a continuous rippling motion. It is so special, I think it is worth describing at length.

For this stroke your partner should be lying flat.

Stand behind them and make initial contact with their face by taking your hands from the throat and sweeping them slowly up over the chin and cheeks, onto the temples and up into the hairline.

Place your hands vertically on the forehead, fingers down towards the nose. As you stroke in an upwards direction, remember to begin your stroke in the air before letting your hands make contact with your partner's skin. Mould your hands to the face and the bridge of the nose, using one hand after another, so that as one stroke is ending the next is beginning in a flowing line of movement. Follow the face around to the sides with this long upward stroke.

Turn your hands so that they are resting horizontally on the forehead, fingers facing each other, and stroke outwards from the centre to the sides of the face. Use only one hand and one finger at a time (i.e. left hand: little finger, fourth finger, third finger, index finger and thumb; then the same with the right hand). Gradually move down the face in this way, out across the cheeks and over the sides of the face.

Circle the left eye with your left hand, using the pads of the index and third fingers placed together; move from the nose, around the cheekbone to the outer face; then with the fingers of your right hand continue over and just above the eyebrow, ending up once again at the nose. You have now made a complete circle around the eye. Now repeat this on the same eye, using just the fourth finger. Finally, do it using just the little finger to describe an entire circle round the eye; move your finger very gently all around the delicate area of the eye socket.

Repeat the entire routine on the right eye, using the fingers of the right hand below it and completing the circle with the fingers of the left hand above the eye.

Now for the skull: for this stroke your partner can be lying down or sitting with their back to you (you will need to be positioned at a higher level).

We have a thin layer of muscle on our skull which can cause headaches when we are anxious. Tension can be relieved by giving the scalp a massage, stroking lightly up from the forehead, over the head and down to the neck. Then, as if you are washing someone's hair, use the fingertips and thumbs to make small circles all over the scalp. The more you move the skin on the scalp, the more you will help the muscles relax. You can then stroke the hair softly and run your fingers through it.

Sandalwood and Frankincense

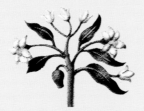

SANDALWOOD oil is obtained from the heartwood of the sandalwood tree. It is one of the oldest known perfume materials, and is commonly used as a blender or fixative.

Much sandalwood comes from India and it is recorded that the emperor Chandragupta Maurya had a daily massage with an oil consisting of aloe, sandalwood and myrrh. The most popular dusting powder among Indian women is *abeer*, which is made from rose petals, sandalwood, aloes, zedoary (a member of the ginger family) and a few grains of civet pounded to a fine powder.

Sandalwood has a powerful, distinctive aroma and has long been an ingredient of religious ritual. It was used in India, mixed with the mortar of temples, and had the additional advantage of keeping white ants at bay.

An ancient Indian prescription for a flawless skin consisted of powdered sandalwood, rape seed and musk boiled in milk. In Vedic times a commonly used cosmetic ointment was *urgujja*, which contained sandalwood powder mixed to a paste with oil of aloe, rose and jasmine.

When disease was not so widely understood as it is today, sandalwood gained a somewhat sinister aura because it was used in the treatment of leprosy. So anyone wearing it as a perfume was regarded with suspicion, especially in the West.

Sandalwood has also been used in the treatment of infections of the urinary tract, especially cystitis and inflammation of the bladder. Made into a paste with water, it works as a cooling agent for skin inflammations and soothes local eruptions. This paste, when mixed with camphor, brings relief from eczema. Applied externally, it has disinfectant properties and acts as a protective layer on the skin, helping keep away pollution and the harmful effects of the sun.

Taken in minute quantities in an infusion of ginger (3 drops to 30 g/1 oz of infusion), sandalwood also acts as an expectorant. Dry sandalwood powder mixed with rosewater is very efficient in controlling prickly heat and on its own is a reliable insecticide. It also helps to bring down a temperature. And if you dust your bookshelves with it, you will keep bookworms at bay!

Sandalwood blends especially well with rose and is often used to extend the (prohibitively expensive) rose. In this case, when oil of roses is being distilled from rose petals, the vapours are received on a mixture of water and sandalwood oil.

FRANKINCENSE, a gum resin found in southern Arabia, was almost as highly prized as myrrh. It was so expensive that in Alexandria, shops where it was sold had to be protected against thieves. It was difficult to gather, for it grew on the steep slopes of hillsides and ravines, and in Arabia only certain tribes were allowed to collect it. Frankincense was linked to the sun and burned at dawn to the sun god Ra. Today it is produced mainly in Iran and Lebanon.

Burned in a fragrancer, or as incense, it creates a sweetish, spicy smell which is very relaxing.

For a pungent bath aroma, add a few drops of essential oil of frankincense mixed with clary sage.

The Neck

With many of us a large part of our tension collects in the neck and upper back, and if the neck muscles are released it has a knock-on effect of relaxing the shoulders and back.

Your partner should be lying flat for this.

Slide both hands (palms up) under the neck, as far down onto the spine as possible, and draw your hands up the neck so that their head lifts a little and the neck is extended. Gently let the head down again. Now draw your hands up the sides of the face and out through the hair.

Put both hands under your partner's head, lift it and gently roll it over to rest on the left side. Starting on the right, use the palms of each hand in turn to stroke up the neck to the face, moulding your hand to the contours of your partner's skin. Gradually work your way around the neck from right to left. You may find that as your hands move slowly from left to right, the head will inadvertently begin rolling from right to left.

You can also do this stroke using one finger at a time (the technique described above under face massage); the sequence is: little finger, fourth finger, third finger, index finger, thumb.

Lift your partner's head and rest it in one hand then, with the other, massage the powerful muscles on either side at the back of the neck.

Let your partner's head down onto the right side; put your left hand sideways just below the base of the skull and glide it down the neck, then encircle the shoulder and glide your fingers back up the neck to just behind the ear, drawing the stroke out through the hair.

A very effective way to massage these two muscles is to have your partner lie face down with their forehead resting on a small rolled-up towel. (This is so that their nose isn't squashed, and they can still breathe!) In this position you can really get a purchase on those powerful muscles at the back of the neck. Use pulling, kneading and rolling strokes to release them.

The Back

If you are massaging a large area of the body such as the back, you will need to put your whole body into the strokes: your hands will be most alive when their movement is an extension of a general bodily flow.

Have your partner lie face down and position yourself behind their head.

Using the entire surface of your hands, place them at the top of the back, fingers pointing in the direction of their bottom. Glide evenly and firmly down either side of the spine, fan out over the hips to the sides of the body and pull up over the ribs. Complete the circle by bringing your hands around the shoulder-blades and up the back of the neck. The first time you do this stroke, as you draw your hands up the back of the neck, extend the movement out through the hair.

Place your thumbs in the furrows on either side of the top of the spine, resting the whole hand on the body. Slide your thumbs firmly down the spine and bring your hands back to the top by sweeping them around, up the sides of the body and over the shoulders.

There is a delicious light stroke, using the index and third fingers of each hand, one hand after the other, which leaves the nerves of the spine tingling. Position yourself to one side of your partner. Placing the index and third fingers of one hand on either side of your partner's spine, run them swiftly all the way down from top to bottom. Just before you reach the bottom, begin the same stroke with your other hand. If you do this several times in quick succession, your partner will feel a wave of tingling sensation rolling down their backbone.

Stand to the left side of your partner's body and reach over to their right side. Beginning at the bottom, draw one hand after the other up the side over the ribs, moving in the direction of the shoulders and moulding the entire hand to curve around the body.

Many people store a lot of tension in their upper back, especially around and between the shoulder-blades. You can work more deeply on this area with kneading and wringing strokes. To lift the shoulder-blade and enable you to gain better access to the muscle which surrounds it, slip one hand under your partner's shoulder and gently place their forearm across their back.

Legs, Arms and Hands

The legs can seem a tough, daunting part of the body to massage. Work separately on the calf and thigh. Positioning yourself to the side of your partner's body, use kneading and wringing strokes on the calf, paying special attention to the powerful muscles on the inside.

The thighs can be highly sensitive and if they are tense they may be ticklish, so you need a firm yet calming stroke here. Glide both hands up from the knees, then around the sides of the thigh and back down again to complete the circle.

For the arms, position yourself to one side. Using kneading strokes, travel from the shoulder all the way down to the wrist.

A gentle form of the 'Chinese burn' which some of us will remember from schooldays is good for releasing the muscles in the upper arm.

Use both hands to stroke all the way down from the shoulder to the wrist. Then lift one of your partner's hands and massage all over the palm with firm thumb circles.

To finish off, hold one of your partner's hands in your own, and rest your other hand on their heart or forehead. Hold this position for some moments.

Chest and Belly

Your partner should be lying on their back. Stand to one side of them. Moving your hands in parallel, stretch your left hand up the side of their body and bring it towards you. At the same time use your other hand to stroke in the opposite direction, horizontally across their body, so that your hands meet and pass each other en route.

Beginning under the rib cage make a large circle around the belly in a clockwise direction. Continue with this stroke, gradually reducing the size of the circle.

Position yourself behind your partner's head. Glide both hands down between the breasts, then spread them out over the lower rib cage and around the sides of the body. Pull up, go around the breasts, and at the armpits rotate your wrists inwards and complete the circle. Then rotate them outwards over the shoulders and back behind the head.

To finish off, place one of your hands between your partner's breasts (fingers pointing down) and the other on their forehead. Hold this position for some moments.

Stand above their head and place both your hands over their ears. As you remove your hands, draw them up onto the head and out gently through the hair.

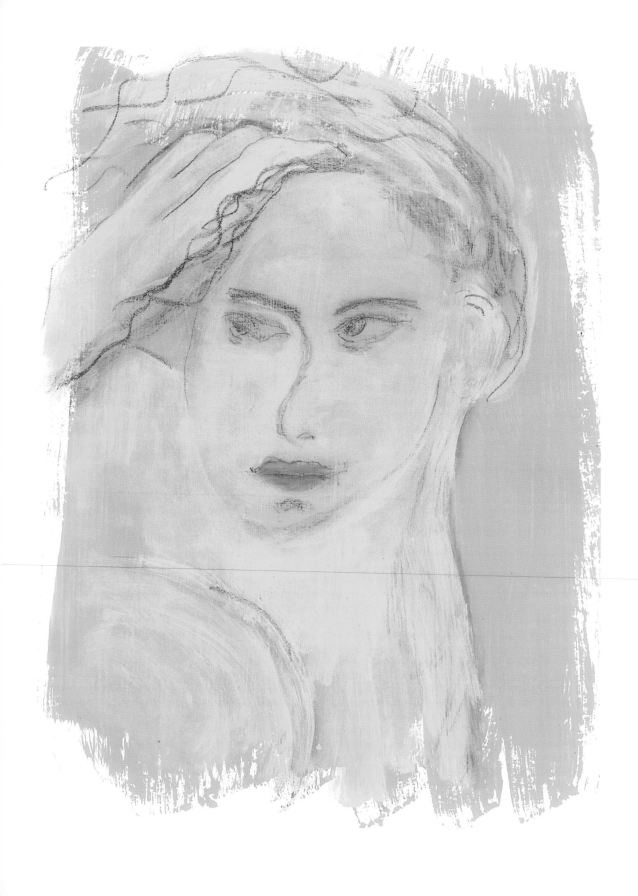

5

The Protective Mask

Who made this maze of uncertainty, this temple of immodesty,
this receptacle of defects, this field sown with a thousand deceits,
this barrier to the gates of heaven, this mouth of the infernal city,
this poison which has the scent of ambrosia, this cord which ties
mortals to the earthly world – in a word, woman?

(The *Kama Sutra*)

A friend of mine who has an Algerian father and a French mother remembers her mother once chiding her for wearing too much make-up. Her father, on the other hand, coming from a culture in which make-up is regarded as a protective mask, had quite the opposite point of view: the more make-up you wear, the more you are shielded from malign spirits and psychic forces. 'I notice', my friend observed, 'that I wear very little in the way of make-up when I'm with friends I trust.'

Many of us understand this feeling of being protected in some nebulous way after we have taken special care in applying cosmetics. This is particularly true in the world of work, where women often have to display much greater energy and confidence than their male colleagues in order to succeed or, sometimes, even be taken seriously.

Beneath the mask, behind the veil, our essential being is hidden and inviolate. As a dancer, I know that when I am on stage, especially if I am giving a solo performance, I am vulnerable to the psychic feedback of my audience. The ritual of putting on make-up before going on stage is an important one and I like to take my time over it in a quiet atmosphere which helps me focus my mind on the performance to come.

Today, when belief in evil spirits is no longer widespread, we still use make-up to exaggerate our sense of ourself, to create ritual and sometimes a sense of drama and fun.

A BRIEF HISTORY OF COSMETICS

In the ancient world, where magic and religion were inextricably intertwined, make-up was used to propitiate the gods. In the great temples it was smeared on the faces of statues, especially on the eyes and lips, and was also used by the officiating priests and priestesses.

The Babylonians coloured their cheeks with red ochre, while the Sumerians used yellow ochre as well as the pernicious white lead on their faces. Using cosmetics to conceal defects, preserve the skin and delight the eye of the onlooker spread westward from ancient Egypt via Greece and Rome.

Our word 'cosmetics' comes from the Greek *kosmetikos*, meaning a person skilled in body decoration. Cosmetics were made in the temple precincts and the raw ingredients for them, the oils and unguents and aromatics, were stored in great jars of onyx and alabaster to prevent them evaporating in the rays of the sun. These highly precious ointments were made from ingredients which had been brought many miles on long overland journeys across the desert. The Romans were very fond of make-up, but when the empire collapsed the use of cosmetics came to be seen as a pagan custom and fell into disrepute.

Medicine was closely linked with magic, as it still is in many parts of the developing world, where the wisdom of linking mental and physical cause and effect has not been lost. Thus it was the therapeutic use of cosmetics which developed before their application as bodily enhancement.

In pharaonic Egypt, children had their eyes heavily made up as a precaution against disease and the glare of the sun (the Egyptian word for 'eye palette' is connected to the verb 'to protect'). The Egyptians painted the faces of their dead to render them more attractive when they entered the afterlife and buried them with beautiful containers full of cosmetics, believing that the next life would be very similar to this one.

Most of our information about the making and use of early cosmetics comes from papyri and inscriptions in the great tombs. The Egyptians did not invent cosmetics but they inherited a tradition which can be traced back to mesolithic times, when the country was inhabited by wandering tribes of hunters and shepherds. Their contribution was to make some ingenious additions to the existing cosmetic repertoire. One was the custom among fashionable women of gilding their nipples and outlining their veins with blue paint. Preparations were (and sometimes still are) made from plant extracts. Seaweed, lichen and mulberry berries were used as dyes and flowers were crushed for their fragrance in hundreds of different combinations.

Women's use of make-up has often attracted criticism from male writers. The Old Testament not only frowned on the use of cosmetics, but on jewellery and hair ornaments as well. Yet while the frivolous use of cosmetics was discouraged, their therapeutic application was accepted. Job named one of his daughters 'Keren Happukh', which meant 'horn of eye paint'.

Until the coming of Christianity, make-up was widely used by women in Europe and the Mediterranean, but the Christian rejection of sensual pleasures led to a decline in their use. In medieval Europe cosmetics became associated with the luxury of the East, which Europeans had come into contact with during the Crusades. It was not until Renaissance times that the use of cosmetics slowly began to gain in popularity. This was initially among the aristocracy who, in their position of power, have never much cared what the religious authorities or the lower classes think of them.

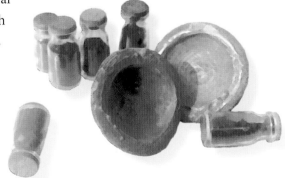

One reason why make-up was frowned on was that it was used by prostitutes. In ancient Greece, prostitutes used thick face powder, dyed their hair blonde and wore bright red lipstick to announce their profession. Sixteenth-century courtesans favoured a pink rouge; so, to dissociate themselves from their 'fallen'

sisters, high-born women favoured the pale, natural if not dead white look. In seventeenth-century Europe black face patches (sometimes a dozen at a time) were worn, cut in the shape of stars, moons and birds. They were made of silk, leather or velvet and helped hide the scars of smallpox to which many fell prey (only milkmaids escaped the scourge, having been naturally vaccinated by catching cowpox as they went about their work).

A day at the steam baths concluded with the careful application of make-up, and *halawa* was sometimes used by older women to give their cheeks a rosy tint. After pulling off the *sukkar* (a lemon and sugar mixture), they pinched and rubbed their cheeks until they were a delicate shade of pink, then added face powder made of cochineal for good measure. Winifred Blackman, who lived in Egypt in the late nineteenth century, tells us that one woman she knew went to the extreme length of applying *halawa* to her cheeks every day as part of her make-up routine.

Perhaps the most exaggerated presentation of a stark white face is that of Japanese women who, traditionally, from the age of 15, used to wear a pale foundation on their skin. They emphasized this effect still further by wearing dark clothes and shaving their eyebrows. In northern Japan there used to be a tradition of lacquering the teeth black and using blue lipstick as a further contrast to the pallor of the face. The lips were sometimes tattooed blue as well, to prevent evil spirits entering the mouth.

Traditional face powder was made from rice flour mixed with egg white. Talcum powder consisted of orris root combined with sandalwood and the roots of lemon grass, which grows abundantly in the sand-dunes of the Sahara.

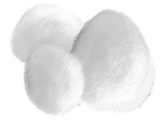

Oranges

A Lemon and Orange Face Mask from India

This face mask uses the peel of 1 lemon and 1 green orange. Green, or unripe oranges are seasonal and can be found in shops specializing in Middle Eastern food. (If unavailable, a lemon can be substituted.) Grind the skins finely and mix them with just enough water to make a paste. Apply this paste to your face. If it's fine weather, lie in the sun for 20 minutes until the paste warms up and seeps into your pores. Wipe off any excess, leaving a coating of natural oils on your skin. This refreshing mask should leave your face glowing and smooth as silk.

An Orange Moisturizer

For a moisturizer, pat fresh orange pulp onto the face, allow it to dry, then rinse off with warm water.

For Healthy Teeth

Orange flower tea can be used as an effective mouthwash, and should be kept refrigerated. Or try pulverized orange peel, with salt as an optional addition, as a toothpaste.

For Greying Hair

An old Arab recipe for restoring colour to greying hair uses the liquid produced by steeping green oranges in olive oil for several weeks.

Pomanders

In many hot countries pomanders are used to keep flies and other insects at bay. They are easily made, using oranges or other thin-skinned citrus fruits. Cover the surface of the

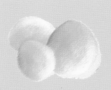

orange skin with whole cloves stuck closely together (if they do not go in easily, pierce the skin with a skewer). Place the cloved orange in a dish containing equal parts of cinnamon, sandalwood and orris root (a traditional fixative). Roll the fruit around in this mixture until it is completely dried out. Alternatively, keep it in a cool, dark place until it has dried. It can then be hung up to keep insects away, or in a cupboard to scent your clothes. Its effect should last for about six months.

White Coffee
Today it has become the fashion in Lebanon to offer guests 'white coffee' (an infusion of orange flower water served in a small coffee cup) after their meal. In Lebanese restaurants you may well be offered a choice of 'black or white coffee'; if you reply, 'white', do not be too surprised when a cup of refreshing sweetened orange flower water is placed in front of you.

OLD COSMETICS STILL IN USE TODAY

In Saudi Arabia you can still find thick, brightly coloured creams made from crushed flowers and powdered stones (including semi-precious ones) together with dried herbs and spices. These are similar to cosmetics used thousands of years ago. The recipes are passed from mother to daughter, with the women modifying them to produce their own favourite fragrance. Iranian women use the highly expensive *sorkhab*, made of rose petals; and Indian women make lipstick out of butter mixed with colouring.

Moroccan women sometimes use a thin solution of *ghassoul* (see page 115) to give their cheeks a pink glow, and in the spice souks you can find little pottery dishes of iron oxide. If you wet the surface with one finger and rub the substance on your lips, the iron oxide will stain them a bright scarlet.

In North Africa beauty spots are painted on the cheeks and on the side and middle of the nose. They are also applied, rather ominously, we may think, in a descending line of dots on both cheeks, to suggest two symmetrical tracks of tears.

MIRRORS OF THE SOUL

Like eye paint is my desire.
When I see you it makes my eyes sparkle.

(Traditional Egyptian song)

Greater symbolism is attached to the eye than to any other part of the body. In Hindu and Buddhist mythology there is a third, or hidden eye, situated in the middle of the forehead; this is the all-seeing eye of spiritual perception, the 'eye of the heart'.

As the symbol of omniscience, the eye possesses great power for good and ill. Throughout the East the concept of the evil eye is a potent one: the belief that if someone wishes you harm all they need do is cast you a malevolent look and bad luck will befall you. Rituals to protect oneself against 'the eye' are legion. In countries surrounding the Mediterranean, necklaces of blue beads on which an eye is inscribed are worn as an active charm against malicious energy. In the Arab world the protective hand of Fatima is daubed on walls and pictures of this hand are also displayed inside the house. You can see hand-of-Fatima charms worn as pendants or hidden inside a little silver case hanging round the neck, and indeed all kinds of jewellery contain talismans against ill fortune. If someone is thought to have been cast a baleful, envious glance, a friend may mutter the single word 'eye' in warning.

Dorina Neave, who lived in Turkey for many years in the late nineteenth century, records a method used to discover the identity of someone who had cast the evil eye: a clove was stuck on the end of a pin and passed through a flame. As it roasted in the fire, the names of suspected individuals were uttered:

when the clove exploded, the culprit was thought to have been found.

Winifred Blackman lived among the Egyptian fellahin (peasants) during the same period. She records that a woman who thought someone had cast the evil eye on her would throw a handful of earth after their departing figure to neutralize the black magic. A more complicated remedy was to find a way of secretly cutting off a small fragment of the suspected person's clothing; it was then placed in a saucer of burning incense and the saucer was brandished in front of the suspect.

Special care is still taken to protect newborn babies from malevolent influences. It is thought that anything that a pregnant woman looks at for any length of time will affect her unborn child, so she may hang pictures of people famous for their beauty and loving disposition around the house. If the mother looks at portraits of these people, it is thought that the child will resemble them. After the baby arrives the hand of Fatima is hung round its neck. Then on the seventh day after the birth, a mixture of onion juice, salt, oil and sometimes kohl is prepared in a coffee cup. A feather is dipped in this paste and passed across the baby's open eyes to make them wide and beautiful.

The ancient Egyptians used a blue eyeliner made from powdered lapis lazuli and soothed their eyes with a solution of ground celery and hemp. Cleopatra painted her upper eyelids blue, the lower ones a brilliant green, and extended the shape of her eyes out to the sides of her face as 'wings', using black galena (powdered grey lead ore).

Eyes were considered the most important part of the body to be emphasized with cosmetics. Although the initial use of eye make-up, like cosmetics in general, was protective (in both the physical and spiritual sense), the realization that it enlarged the eyes and made them appear more beautiful no doubt gave rise to its use for purely decorative purposes. Originally eye make-up was kept in shells, then in manufactured containers of great workmanship fashioned from ivory, silver or wood. Some of these containers were made out of different types of glass according to the season of the year. It is still possible to find beautiful silver *makhallas* (see illustration on opposite page), kohl-containers stoppered with ornate applicators fashioned in the shape of palm trees and other natural forms.

Among the gifts traditionally given by an Indian groom to his bride is a box of make-up including a kohl-container and *soorma* (a type of kohl). When they marry she adds to her usual make-up with a line of gold and silver dots encircling the eye socket, and may rub gold glitter all over her body too.

In Turkey and Iran it was once considered beautiful to paint the eyebrows in a single line across the bridge of the nose. Julia Pardoe, visiting Turkey a century ago, wrote of 'this dreadful custom of joining the eyebrows artificially across the nose, by which mistaken habit I have seen many a really pretty face terribly disfigured.'

KOHL

A friend of mine who lived in Morocco for several years reminisced: 'When a sandstorm was on its way, we would hear a man come riding past the house on his horse, blowing a trumpet, calling out for us to put on our kohl to protect our eyes from the dust.'

The literal meaning of kohl is 'to brighten the eyes'. Kohl is used throughout the East as a cosmetic and as protection against eye ailments and is traditionally applied just inside the eyelids. As black is known to absorb the light, kohl was used initially to protect against the glare of the sun. It was also used to help prevent eye disease, by repelling the tiny flies which transmit disease and inflammation, and to prevent the delicate skin around the eye socket from becoming dry and cracked. However, the belief that all varieties of kohl are beneficial is not entirely justified. The kohl used in ancient Babylon is thought to have been made of arsenic, a white metallic substance which turns black on exposure to the air. One variety of kohl in ancient Egypt contained ants' eggs and lead. Recently, Indian and Persian *soormas* were found to contain lead sulphate, though it continues to be used.

Kohl is made from different substances in different countries. In the past the flesh of a lemon was scooped out and the skin filled with plumbago and burnt copper; this was placed on a charcoal brazier until it became carbonized; it was then pounded with a pestle and mortar. Little pieces of pulverized coral, pearls and ambergris were added, with the final addition of charred bats' wing moistened with rosewater.

Today kohl is made out of pulverized antimony or olive stones (Morocco), lead (India) and the soot from various nuts, seeds and gum resins. In the Egyptian countryside it is made by combining sunflower soot and charred almond shells perfumed with frankincense. Scented kohl made from labdanum incense is obtained by throwing a piece of this gum into an incense burner and collecting the ascending smoke in the form of soot, by holding a plate above the smoke.

Kohl is applied with a wooden, silver or ivory stick, moistened with water or rosewater before being dipped in the kohl pot. It is applied right inside the eye by taking the stick from the nose outwards, closing the eye over it as it is drawn towards the outer eye in a straight line.

To Make the Eyes Sparkle

A common method of making the eyes more brilliant is to use an infusion of feverfew or chrysanthemum. Belladonna (literally, 'beautiful woman') was once widely used throughout the Mediterranean to artificially enlarge the pupils, but it had a harsh effect on the eyes and has been replaced now by bathing the eyes with an infusion of the herb eyebright or soaking pads of lint and placing them over the closed eyelids.

A Persian remedy for puffiness and bags under the eyes is to use a daily compress of eucalyptus oil and wheat extract.

Pads of cotton wool soaked in cucumber juice, placed on the closed eyelids, will soothe and cool the eyes. It has been suggested that squeezing a little cucumber juice directly into the eyes has a toning effect. But I wouldn't advise this, for it is easy to inadvertently squeeze a miniscule piece of cucumber flesh into your eye, which will cause a lot of pain until it works its way out.

To Darken the Eyelashes and Eyebrows

Here is an old Persian remedy, used daily, to enhance dark eyelashes: boil up walnut leaves until they are reduced to a thick, dark, coffee-like liquid. Moisten the eyelashes and eyebrows with this liquid.

THE EYE AND THE VEIL

Three things alone
Prevent her black eyes saying yes:
Fear of the unknown, and horror of the known,
And her own loveliness.

(The Thousand and One Nights)

The eye has always been considered a chief erogenous zone. In certain Muslim countries, women are compelled by law to cover not only the eyes but the entire face behind an all-enveloping black veil. In others, a woman's eye is the only part of the face visible, and thus assumes even greater significance.

Women have often used their veils to draw attention to their faces. More than one nineteenth-century traveller to the Middle East, where veils had become fashionable, commented on ways in which a woman would skilfully adjust and manipulate her face veil in order to convey a message, in much the same way that European society women used their fans.

Women have devised many different styles of veil which turn them into attractive items of clothing. An Iranian friend once gave me an old face veil of a type used in her grandmother's day by fashionable women at parties. Attached behind the head, it was made of black velvet embroidered with loops of silver beads and allowed the observer to see something of the face behind the delicately glittering filigree of beading.

Certain types of veils, which cover the face while allowing the eyes to remain visible, have the effect of bringing the eyes into greater prominence than if the entire face were hidden. Old bedouin face veils, which are covered in silver coins and dangling strings of amber, are items of sinister beauty. They are tied behind the head and fitted over the face so that they hang down onto the chest. The first

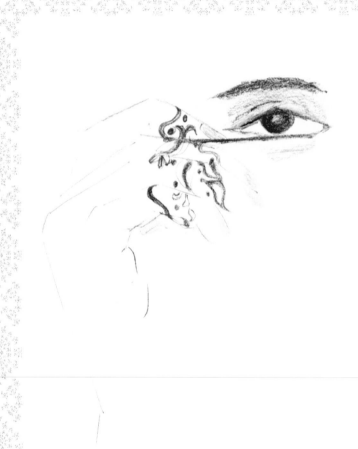

time I tried one on, in connection with a performance I was devising, I found it so heavy and suffocating that it was hard to move my head while wearing it.

The origin of female veiling is hotly debated today among liberal Muslims, who consider it a shameful custom which should, by now, have disappeared. Some Arabs state that the custom originated in Persia, while Iranians claim the opposite. Certain authorities point out that in any case there is evidence that it was pre-Islamic; they say its role was not initially intended to deprive women of either their freedom or their identity, though in time this became the case. It is true that the veil has a practical, protective aspect, and in the desert there are tribes of both men and women who veil to prevent sand entering the nose and mouth, as well as to shield the head from the sun. However, it is instructive to see how an item of clothing with so many positive, practical uses has, over many years, been hijacked as a means of controlling the female sex.

In ancient Assyria and Babylon the veil was used as a symbol of rank. Slaves and prostitutes were forbidden to cover their faces, and so the veil became a sign of both the free-born and the wealthy. Because wearing a veil has high social standing today, in poor Muslim countries such as Yemen the custom has developed whereby immigrant workers returning home veil their wives as a sign of their own rise in the social hierarchy. In this way, women living in rural areas who formerly moved about unveiled without any fear of being molested now find themselves under pressure to hide their faces and thus proclaim their untouchability.

Verse 24 of the Qur'an enjoins a woman to dress modestly and not display her charms. In time this verse came to be interpreted as meaning that a woman should cover her entire face. But in the first century of Islam there were leading women sages, poets and rulers who did not cover their faces. The veil is thought to have been adopted by women as a means of self-protection against the visual aggression of men, and it is partially used today with this intention in Egypt. There, although it is not required by law, women are increasingly covering their heads, as in the past; a decision which owes much to social pressure and the belief that a woman may be dishonoured if a man merely looks at her lustfully. However there are many Egyptian women who continue to wear heavy make-up and large earrings, to compensate for feeling obliged to cover their hair.

Wearing veils which completely cover the face forces women to fumble about beneath them in order to eat and drink, and some bedouin face veils have removable sections for freedom of movement. Otherwise, in order to eat, a woman has to go through the business of lifting the veil which covers her nose and mouth and quickly passing her food beneath it.

Today in Saudi Arabia female children may be veiled as early as 4 years old, and there are women who keep their veils on even when they are in bed asleep. In the capital, Riyadh, local government officials spend a considerable amount of time dealing with complaints from men who accuse their male neighbours of attempting to catch a glimpse of their wives over the walls of adjacent houses.

Throughout history, men have invented rules and taboos to deal with that which they fear. By a cruel twist of fate, a device which was originally used by women for their own protection against men who sought to subjugate them has become a means whereby women continue to collude in their own oppression.

Compelled by law to keep her face covered at all times, a woman living in a strict Islamic country may live out her entire existence without ever feeling the rays of the sun on her face; an anonymous figure so devoid of identity that even when she dies her veil may remain in place, as much a part of her body as her skin itself.

BODY DESIGNS

In black Africa and Upper Egypt self-mutilation, in the form of tribal scarification, indicates a sense of identity, of belonging to the group. It is also used to draw attention to a beautiful part of the body. Dots and lines are cut into the body and ash is rubbed into them so that they stand out in a braille of raised scars, messages which can be interpreted by touch. They are often made around an admired part of the body, such as the belly or the breasts.

The same is true of tattoos. In Africa and the Middle East they were used in the past to distinguish criminals, the poor, outlaws and slaves. In ancient Egypt the practice of tattooing seems to have been reserved for women, especially those of low status such as prostitutes and entertainers. Yet tattooing, like cosmetic care in general, also possesses a powerful magical significance. It has been found on mummies of priestesses and dancers from the second millennium BC, discovered in the temple of Hatshepsut. When a slave converted to

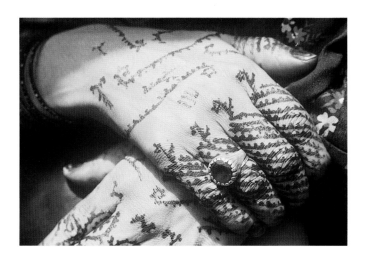

Islam, he or she was instantly freed from slavery; because of this, the practice of tattooing was forbidden under Islam. It has nonetheless continued down to the present day in North Africa and Yemen, as well as among the bedouin. There, women tattoo their chins, hands, foreheads and sometimes between the breasts with patterns and symbols from pre-Islamic days. The ritual significance of these designs was partly designed to be therapeutic; but the original meaning of the patterns has largely been lost with the passage of time. In tattooing a pattern is pricked out on the skin with a needle, and these punctures are then rubbed with milk or lampblack mixed with oil or water.

Winifred Blackman recollected that tattooers used to parade the Egyptian streets alerting people to their presence. They would travel to the local souk and sit under a tree with their designs displayed all around them. The operation often resulted in a mild fever and a swelling of the tattoed area, which eventually died down.

Tattoos on the back of the hand or wrist were said to strengthen this part of the body. A dot on the side of the nose was thought to cure toothache, while a mark on either side of the temples – perhaps in the shape of a bird – was a cure for headaches. If a woman had lost several children in succession, she would have the next baby to survive tattooed with a small dot in the middle of its forehead and on the outer edge of the left ankle in the belief that the baby's life would then be safeguarded. Coptic Christians often had a cross tattooed in the middle of their wrists.

The custom of applying designs to the surface of the body, rather than cutting them into the skin, has lost none of its popularity, and becomes more pronounced the further south we travel into Africa. In a sense this elaborate body painting takes the place of clothes in terms of self-adornment, especially in hot climates, and it can look extremely beautiful.

In many societies those who lack a sense of self-worth or identity take the least care of the image they present to the outside world, so body painting is intimately linked with a woman's self-esteem.

Henna

One of the most poignant sights I have seen on my travels was in India, in the ruins of a temple in Rajasthan. All around the lintel were the imprints of women's palms which had been dipped in henna, then pressed into the walls around the entrance. These women had been about to commit suttee and their final act before throwing themselves on their husbands' funeral pyres was to leave behind them this sign of their passing.

Henna can be said to play an almost mystical role in tradition. Among Moroccan Berber women it is worn to ward off evil spirits, and in some Arab countries sacks of henna leaves form part of a bride's dowry.

The henna shrub probably originated in Persia but it now grows throughout the Middle East, Africa and Asia. It has pink and cream coloured flowers which produce blue-black berries. Some say the best varieties come from Iraq and Saudi Arabia. Henna grown in Iran gives a deep colour, while Egyptian and Moroccan henna produces a more orange dye. Staining the skin with henna designs is one of the most arresting and beautiful customs in terms of body painting. It was a custom in ancient Egypt, where women used henna to tint the breasts and navel a rosy hue. It was also used to dye the hair and nails of mummies. In the twelfth century the Mughals introduced henna to India, where it rapidly became popular.

Today henna has numerous uses in the Middle East and North Africa. Nubian women place the leaves under their armpits as a deodorant. Mixed with acacia leaves, henna relieves sore hands and feet. Mixed with vinegar and applied to the brow, it is thought to relieve headaches and other heat-induced ailments.

When someone is running a temperature, or if the heat is especially fierce, henna paste is used as a body-cooling agent. In this case it is applied to the palms and soles of the feet, giving them a rosy stain. It is also used as a hair conditioner, and when it is rinsed out of the hair a little of the diluted solution is rubbed on the cheeks as rouge.

The most popular uses of all are as a hair dye and to decorate the body on special occasions, such as the post-Ramadan religious festival, *'Id*.

The henna ceremony preceding a marriage is the most important of a young girl's wedding preparations. It is an occasion of much merriment, with singing and dancing, eating and drinking. The bride cannot move, of course, or

> the henna would smudge, so her friends feed her while she
> sits on her cushions like a princess, waiting patiently for the
> patterns to dry.

HENNA PAINTING

Several summers ago in Morocco I had my hands and feet painted with henna. It took a couple of hours for Amina to finish her task and she applied herself with concentration, using swift, practised strokes. It is the custom to offer the henna painter tea and cakes, so after Amina had finished my feet we paused for some refreshment. Lying there with my hands and feet held out to the sun, I couldn't help wondering by what process of trial and error this custom had been invented and refined. Whoever was it who discovered that, if you pound henna leaves, mix them with liquid into a paste, then paint your hair or body with it, a deep-stained colour will result? And how did they figure out that if you apply certain other substances after you've done this it will help fix the colour?

The touch of the dark green henna with its delicious earthy smell was cool on my skin and I watched with fascination as a garden of tendrils and flowers took shape, sketched with perfect sureness of touch by Amina. By the time she had finished the sun was beginning to go down, and my hands and feet looked as if they were covered in little black lacy gloves and socks. She ended by painting my nails, and I remembered having been told by another Moroccan woman why henna was preferred to nail varnish. She told me that using varnish contravenes Islamic cleanliness rituals. 'Varnish creates a barrier which water can't penetrate, so you can't clean your nails properly,' she said. With henna, on the other hand, the nails are simply coated and water can seep through.

When Amina was done with the painting she took a ball of cotton wool, dipped it in a jar of amber-coloured liquid and dabbed it all over her patterns, leaving them glistening black. As I lifted one of my hands to examine its black lacy glove, I caught a strong whiff of garlic.

For important occasions it is not unusual to paint the hands, feet and

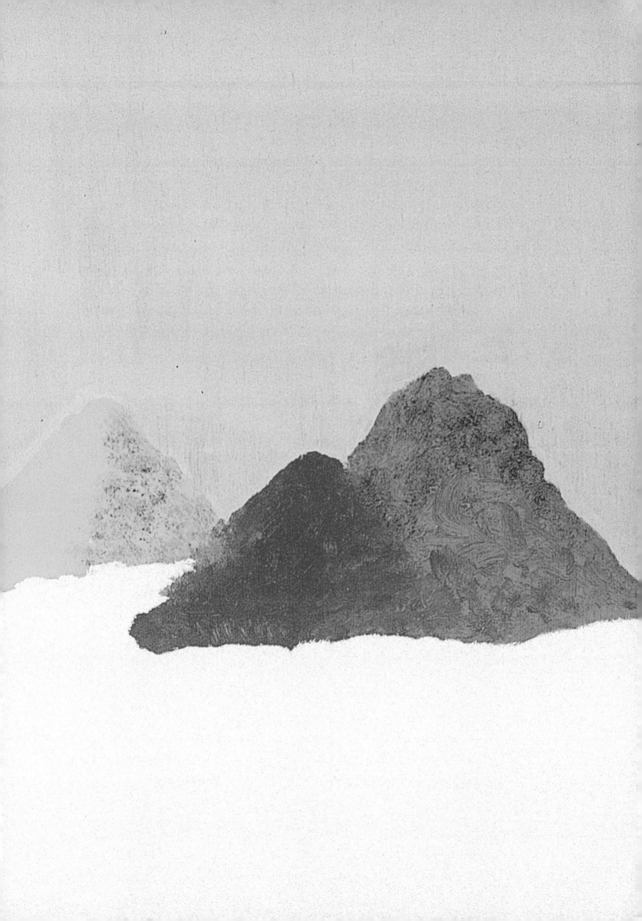

sometimes the entire arms and legs with patterns of extraordinary intricacy and beauty. Most significant of all is the henna painting before a wedding. Depending on the family finances, wedding celebrations in many Middle Eastern and Asian countries can last for anything from three to seven days. On the night before the wedding the women have a party and decorate the bride, who becomes a human canvas for the skills of the henna painter. According to how long they have been left on before the henna is scraped off, these designs will gradually fade over a period of time, usually one to three weeks, as the top layers of skin are worn away. Henna painting is particularly popular in North Africa, Yemen, Bahrain, Sudan and India (where it is known as *mehendi*). Depending on the country and whether it is a rural or urban area, henna is applied either in a smooth coat or in elaborate patterns. These patterns vary from town to town. A Moroccan woman, for example, can tell if someone is from Fez or Marrakesh simply by looking at the henna patterns on her hands.

In Tunisia simple geometric designs are favoured, while in Morocco and India the hand looks as if it is wearing a delicate lace glove. Scallops, stars, crescents, flowers, fish scales, elaborate circular mandalas . . . the variety of designs is unending. The meaning of these patterns, if it ever existed, has been lost over time, and among educated Westernized women the tradition is no longer as widespread as it once was. But it is still by no means uncommon to see a bride dressed in a white, Western-style wedding dress, with her hands henna-stained in the old way. In Abha (Saudi Arabia) a bride has henna patterns all the way up her arms, which, combined with the glorious plaits of flowers adorning her hair and falling over her shoulders, creates an effect of dazzling beauty.

Today you can buy throw-away transfers of these designs, which makes the process easier, though not nearly as enjoyable as seeing a gifted artist at work on your body!

A young Indian woman I spoke to laughed with delight when she recalled the henna night of her wedding: 'I couldn't do anything for myself. I lay on the sofa with my feet on cushions and my arms out. The other girls had to feed me, they had to do everything for me! I left it on overnight so the colour would come out stronger. Men just love the smell of henna on a woman's body!'

Preparation and Painting with Henna

As in the preparation of henna for the hair (see page 116), the powdered leaves are mixed with water or lemon juice (lemon juice acts as a fixative) and brought to a paste-like consistency. Traditionally, the darker the shade, the more beautiful it is thought to be.

If you want a deep hue – a burgundy or dark brown – then mix the henna with brewed tea or coffee instead of water. To create an intense, near-black colour, pulverized indigo leaves can be added.

If you want just an expanse of colour, rather than a pattern, cup a large lump of henna paste in your hand in such a way that the lines on your palm are not covered with the henna. Later, when the henna is scraped off, these lines will stand out as they do when a palmist takes your hand print.

You can also smooth henna paste on the pads of the fingers or on the nails of the hands and feet.

Henna designs are traditionally applied to the skin using a fine wooden or silver stick. Some people use a plastic cone or an icing-sugar applicator, squeezing out the henna in a fine thread through the nozzle, and you can also use cottonbuds.

Nowadays some professional henna-painters use a syringe with the end of the needle blunted. Applying henna in patterns by hand takes quite a while, so even if you only want your feet or the backs of your hands decorated, be prepared for a couple of hours lying around waiting for it to dry.

After the patterns have been applied, dab them periodically with a piece of cotton wool soaked in a mixture of lemon juice and sugar to help them set. Sometimes garlic is also added to this solution. If you want a really deep colour, you can sleep with the henna on (you will have to wear socks or gloves unless you want it to be smeared all over your sheets by the morning!). When you scrape off the henna, rub olive oil into your skin to help condition it and deepen the colour.

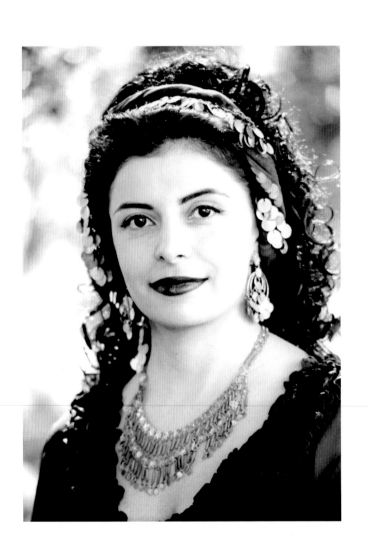

6

Hair

A saffron-scented perfume trails
Before the senses,
Even now her fragrance lingers.
The folds of her hair redolent as musk when the pod is opened
Reaching out to touch it, even a stuffy nose is overcome.

('Alqamah bin 'Abdah, *al-Mufaddaliyah Ode*)

Our distant ancestors interpreted the streaming tail of a comet as the long hair of the goddess who had created all things. This, they thought, was the last we would see of her before she left us to our destiny.

In terms of its magical and symbolic significance, hair has been written about more than any other part of the human body. Its prodigious powers are such that it carries on growing even after we die and recent studies have shown that sexual activity (or even the mere expectation of it) is enough to stimulate the growth of our hair.

It has been remarked that we tend to cut or in some way change our hairstyle at a significant point of change in our life. In the 1960s Western men grew their hair as a sign of protest against the establishment and, most noticeably, against the Vietnam war. Indeed, in the sixties hair assumed such significance as a badge of youth that a theatre show was named for it and songs written in celebration of it!

Once upon a time it was only the ruling classes who were permitted to have long hair. The poor were compelled to keep theirs cropped, and even in recent times the first thing that happened to a man when he was sent to gaol was to cut him down to size by cropping his hair.

According to one theory, our words for king or ruler – shah, tsar and kaiser – all stem from a root meaning 'long-haired'.

In ancient Egypt, the shaved head of the pharaoh was considered sacred and was hidden from the sight of the public under a wig. These wigs, which also had the practical use of protecting the wearer against the sun, were made of human hair combined with vegetable fibre, plaited grass and black sheep's wool, all held in place with beeswax. In time these confections grew highly stylized. False beards were adopted as a sign of power in men and women alike. (Queen Hatshepsut used a gilded beard on ceremonial occasions, when she needed to assert her authority.) Tall wigs known as macaronies were popular in eighteenth-century Europe and signified the wearer's high social rank (they were, however, so tall and heavy that they occasionally caused fatal abscesses on the temples).

Even now long hair, whether real or false, retains an echo of its association with power, and anyone wondering why English judges still wear long grey wigs in session need look no further than this for an explanation.

HAIR IN FOLKLORE AND MYTHOLOGY

Your hair, let down and loose,
Like a soft shore, inhabited
With musk, perfume and incense,
Leads me on
To an enchanted cave.

(Hisham Ali Hafi)

For thousands of years, hair has been the subject of folklore, mythology and religious writings throughout the world. The writhing snakes of the Medusa's black tresses are a potent symbol of the feared aspect of female power. From Indian tantric sagas, warning that a catastrophe would occur if a woman let down her hair, to the medieval belief that tempests were the result of witches unbraiding their locks, hair has long symbolized the dangerous power of women.

During the witch hunts of the Middle Ages, those unfortunate women who were convicted and condemned to death for their supposedly magical powers were 'purified' before being burnt at the stake by having their hair shorn off.

When Delilah chopped off Samson's locks she robbed him not only of his hair but also his manly strength. The three male-centred religions which have dominated our world, Judaism, Christianity and Islam, all place great importance on the erotic significance of a woman's hair and each has devised laws relating to it. St Paul thundered at women to cover their hair if they wanted to embrace Christianity; only in this way, he said, could they prove their modesty and devotion to God. By covering her hair, a nun demonstrates that she has renounced her human sexuality and become a symbolic bride of Christ. As already mentioned, Hasidic Jewish brides shave their hair and wear a wig, to remove the magical properties of their natural hair. Meanwhile strict Muslims are so fearful of the power of female hair that they demand that women cover their heads and that every single hair on the body, including pubic hair, is removed. (And while we are on the subject, it is recorded that medieval knights sometimes took a lock of their sweetheart's pubic hair into battle as a love token.) Originally, the habit of giving a lover a lock of one's hair to wear in a locket round the neck was not only a sentimental gesture, but could be seen as a dangerous one as well. For it was well known that magicians could use a lock of someone's hair to cast a spell on them.

Our hair is so imbued with our intrinsic nature or life-force that analysing it can reveal a great deal about our state of health. In certain African countries people still hide their hair clippings so that sorcerers cannot use them to cast spells; and in the past, American Indians who scalped their victims used the power of this hair to decorate their shields.

But in certain cultures hair has another significance and is used to honour the dead. There are East African warriors who make the sacrifice of shaving their hair when one of their tribe dies, thus stripping themselves of an important aspect of their beauty. Similarly, in imperial Japan a woman cut her hair when her husband died so that he could take it with him into the next world.

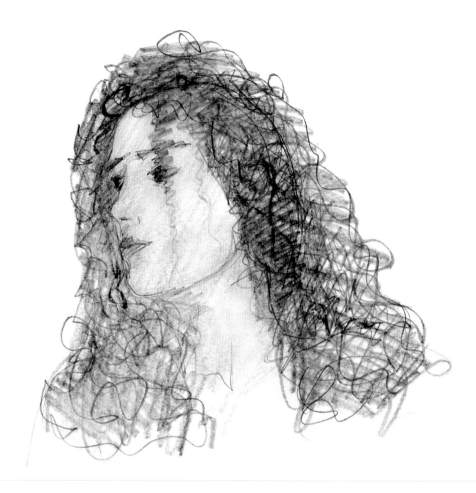

HAIR IN HISTORY

The racy overtones of blonde hair can be traced back to the days of classical Greece, when it was the custom for prostitutes to dye their hair yellow or to wear a blonde wig. In Rome this applied to red as well as blonde hair.

Fashion in hair style and colour ebbs and flows through the ages. In neo-Babylonian times curly fringes were popular and during the Abbasid period cropped hair for women was considered a sign of beauty. The Assyrians oiled and perfumed their hair and wigs and developed elaborate hairdressing to the exclusion of nearly every other cosmetic art.

Cleaning the hair by immersing it in water is a relatively recent custom. In fact the word 'shampoo' comes from a Hindu word meaning 'to knead or rub'. Old recipes for shampoo are based on powders brushed repeatedly through the hair until all the grease and dirt have been banished; sometimes floral and herbal rinses mixed with oil were used, and one old recipe advises a mixture of opium and rose in cedar oil.

In the ancient world, hair was cleaned frequently and lightened with saffron. Cassia was massaged into the scalp mixed with olive oil, to keep lice at bay. (The oil prevented the penetration of oxygen and in this way suffocated the lice.) Cassia, which contains tannic acid, was used to dye the hair and to produce a blackish-green hue.

From Cleopatra's time we find recipes for preventing hair loss which include lion fat and arsenic; greying hair was treated with a concoction that included the blood of a black bull, though with what results we can only surmise.

Follies of the past include the sixteenth-century Venetian habit of sitting out in the sun with the hair drenched in caustic soda, which caused sunstroke. During this period red hair was so popular that English women used to apply a mixture of saffron and sulphur powder to their hair, with the result that they often suffered headaches, nosebleeds and nausea. In the seventeenth century lead combs were popular as a means of dyeing the hair black; needless to say, kidney failure and lead poisoning were sometimes the result of using these combs.

Fashion in hair colour, though, has a lot to do with the universal longing for what we don't have, as well as our liking for change.

In her first book of memoirs, *The Dancer of Shamahka*, the dancer Armen Ohanian gave the following description of a visit to the steam baths as a young girl in Persia:

First the bathers soaped our hair and left it for some time in foamy turbans on our heads. When the soap was washed away the hair was dipped in henna and left wrapped in reddening cloths. After the henna, which strengthens the roots, women rinsed the hair for an hour and covered it with curdled milk, which nourishes the scalp. After another interval came another hour of rinsing and an hour of drying and combing. Then the hair was dipped in rosewater and braided . . .

In India corn meal is used as a traditional dry shampoo. In many parts of the East cleaning the hair does not necessarily include the addition of water, especially in countries where water is scarce. In fact it has been found that too much washing with water and modern shampoos (many of which contain harsh detergents) robs the hair of its natural protective oils. (It is because of this that we need to use conditioners.)

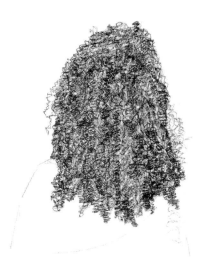

A Dry Shampoo

One method of dry cleaning the hair is to cover a brush with muslin onto which you have sprinkled rose or other floral water. If you give your hair a good brushing, forcing the bristles through the material, you will bring out the dirt. The amount of dirt which is transferred to the brush shows just how effective this method can be. When dry shampoos are thoroughly brushed out they leave the hair gleaming, and help boost its health by not washing out its protective acid mantle.

Pre-wash Conditioners

For dry hair: soak your hair in warm olive oil and wrap it in a hot towel for a minimum of 20 minutes. Rinse with cold water. Shampoo.

For oily hair: mash bananas into your hair and leave for 15 minutes. Shampoo.

For dark hair: yoghurt is a good pre-shampoo conditioner.

Shampoos

In Tahiti women wash their black hair with sandalwood-scented coconut oil. In southern Iraq and the Gulf, a simple shampoo is made out of the leaves of the cidra tree. They are dried, ground to a powder and steeped in water to make a thin, glutinous liquid. (According to ancient belief the cidra tree was sacred to the female deity. Woe betide anyone who cut it down, in which case they could expect to have ten years' bad luck.)

An old Persian shampoo: boil the leaves and roots of nettle, wild marjoram and sage.

A high-protein shampoo: separate the yolk and white of an egg, whisk the white and fold the two together. Massage into the hair and leave it on for a few minutes. Rinse off with tepid water (not warm, unless you want to make scrambled eggs on your head).

Aloe Vera

Aloe vera is used in the Caribbean as a shampoo; cut directly from the plant, it creates a good lather and has a viscous, slippery texture. It adds sheen to hair and also acts as a partial sunscreen. Allow it to dry on the hair then rinse it out.

Rinses

Hair rinses using essential oils keep the hair shiny and full of life.

For dark hair: combine 3 drops of rosemary, 1 drop of rosewood and geranium and 1 l (2 pt) of water.

For fair hair: combine 2 drops of camomile and 1 drop of lemon with water. Shake well to disperse the oils.

Dandruff

A friend who had a problem with dandruff accidentally dropped a bottle of jasmine essential oil in the bath one day while running it. Luckily (for jasmine is one of the costliest oils!) there had only been a little bit left in the bottle, though it was a great deal more than the few drops you would normally use in the bath. A couple of days later my friend reported in amazement that his dandruff had miraculously cleared up!

Dandruff can sometimes result when the shampoo is not washed out thoroughly.

Almond oil is a good general remedy and the heavier olive oil is said to be a miracle cure for dandruff.

Another treatment is to beat 2 egg yolks in 115 ml (390 fl. oz) warm water and massage into the scalp. Leave the eggs on for 10 minutes. Rinse off and then rinse again with 2 teaspoons of vinegar in 225 ml (760 fl. oz) of cool water.

For cradle cap (scaly scalp) in babies: use sweet almond oil, warmed by placing the bottle in a pan of hot water.

Oil Conditioners

Contrary to what we may think, using oil on the hair will not leave you with matted hair, but it must be applied to the scalp rather than the hair itself. Leave it on for half an hour or more and your scalp will be less dry and flaky; it will also give your hair a wonderful sheen and bounce.

Jojoba oil is another good conditioner for dry scalps. Or use a combination of lavender, camomile and geranium. In India the scalp is regularly treated with oil to prevent the build-up of dead cells: almond, jasmine, clove, rose and orange oil are all used, as too is henna.

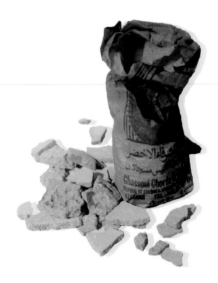

Ghassoul

The most effective hair conditioner I have ever come across, including all the Western products I've tried over the years, is Moroccan *ghassoul* (from *ghassala*, meaning 'to clean'). I first tried it when I was given some by a friend who had lived in Morocco for many years. While I was sitting there with the towel wrapped round my head she remarked casually that it was also a good hair straightener. As my hair is permed I was alarmed, for this was not at all the effect I wanted! But after I'd washed it out and my hair was dry I was delighted to find that the *ghassoul* had had quite the opposite effect. My hair had been transformed beyond belief; it was soft and springy and looked, if anything, twice as curly as before. And it now had the wonderful rosy, earthy smell of the *ghassoul*. Like henna, *ghassoul* is messy to use – you can find Western preparations which include it as one of their ingredients but the effect, needless to say, isn't the same as using pure *ghassoul* from the souk.

Ghassoul is a mixture of pounded moss, rose petals and herbs mixed with water. Women mould it into bricks and leave it out on the roof to dry in the sun. You can buy it at the spice souk in lumps which you then pulverize in a pestle and mortar; you can also buy it in the form of thin, slate-like slivers. Reconstituted with hot water into a paste, it can be used as a conditioner before shampooing the hair. After applying it, wrap your hair in a plastic cap and warm towel and leave it on for around 20 minutes to do its work.

(Ghassoul is also good for cleaning ceramic surfaces; when you rinse it off your hair, you can give the basin a good swill round with the remaining mixture before it disappears down the plughole.)

Today women are increasingly finding that they develop an allergic reaction to the powerful chemical dyes used in hair salons. There is no doubt that chemical dyes not only damage the hair but, when applied externally to the body, may seep into the skin and cause a harmful reaction. Doctors often advise pregnant women not to use these chemical preparations, for fear of harming their unborn baby, and more women are turning to natural preparations than ever before.

Henna has been tested and proved benign, though some henna products which are designed to take speedy effect may contain aniline dye or metallic salts to speed up the process. A natural product always takes longer, but if you can make the time, this can be a benefit; it can enable you to sit round and relax with friends and make a social occasion of it. However, henna is not best suited for permed hair as it interferes with the waving bonds, so use it before, not after, you have had a perm.

Dyeing the Hair with Henna

Iranian henna will dye the hair a deep red; Egyptian and Moroccan henna give more of an orange shade. For a less intense red or a darker colour mix in a little strong coffee. Or use walnut oil to soften the red and give a browner shade to the hair. When using henna on grey hair, an old tradition is to add tea.

Wash your hair before applying henna. The longer you leave it on, the deeper will be the resulting colour. In the Middle East women often apply it in the evening and leave it on overnight, wrapped tightly in muslin, then wash it off the next day.

Like any natural substance, henna is messy to use. It stains anything it touches, so use rubber gloves when applying it and if any falls on your skin wipe it off quickly, unless you want a red face! As a precaution, apply some moisturizing cream around your hairline and ears.

Prepare the henna by mixing a sufficient quantity to make a smooth paste (not too thick) with 200 ml (680 fl. oz) of boiling water. Henna takes time to work and the addition of a teaspoon of lemon juice or vinegar will release the dyeing agent in the henna and accelerate the process. Leave the henna mixture to cool. If your hair is very dry you may like to add a beaten egg to it.

Separate the hair into sections (if you have long hair you can hold it back with clips) and working from the back of the head to the front, apply it with a brush, beginning at the roots. To ensure that your hair is evenly coated, you can twist each strand as you apply the henna.

Wrap your head in muslin, a plastic shower cap or an old scrap of material which you don't mind getting stained. If you have dark hair you will need to leave the henna on for several hours, so it's a good idea to do the henna first and then go on to any other body treats you have in mind.

Rinse out the henna thoroughly, combing it through the hair with a wide-toothed comb. Finish off with a shampoo and conditioner.

Other Hair-colouring Agents

In Iran a paste of indigo and water is applied, to obtain the blue-black hue which is considered most beautiful there.

For dark hair, use the juice of a lemon mixed with a cup of strong black coffee; alternatively use the cooking water left over after boiling up beetroot.

An infusion of sage is a safe, reliable rinse and can be used with tea leaves left in the pot. Place the tea leaves together with a handful of dry sage leaves in a jug filled with 500 ml (1 pt) of boiling water. Leave for an hour, strain and apply to the hair after washing.

The most effective hair darkener is walnut oil, but it must be used with care. It will stain the skin, so wear rubber gloves to protect the hands and apply it with cotton wool.

For fair hair, use a camomile rinse consisting of 2 tablespoons of dried camomile flowers steeped in 600 ml (1¼ pt) hot water and left to cool.

Cedarwood and Myrrh

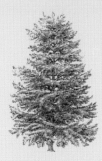

CEDARWOOD. Among the most highly prized oils was cedarwood from the cedars of Lebanon. These long-vanished forests of trees renowned for their beauty were plundered to such an extent in the building of Solomon's Temple in Jerusalem (which was made largely of cedarwood) that they never recovered. The Egyptians believed cedarwood was imperishable and could preserve forever anyone enclosed within it, hence it was much in demand for funerals and embalming.

In the ancient world there were many royal palaces built entirely of cedarwood, which owed its attraction to its insect-repellent qualities as well as its sweet, resiny scent. The Temple of Diana at Ephesus, one of the Seven Wonders of the ancient world, caught fire in 356 BC and one can imagine the aromatic scent of its flames as its towering columns burnt to the ground.

Today's cedarwood oil comes from North Africa and is known for its antiseptic qualities. It is used to ameliorate catarrh and respiratory ailments and in the treatment of skin complaints, and has a warm, sweet smell when burned as incense.

MYRRH was one of the most prized aromatics in the ancient world, and before the use of animal fixatives was the sole substance which could provide a strong, long-lasting fragrance. Myrrh was used throughout the Middle East in embalming and was placed among clothes and linen to perfume them with its strong, resinous scent. Little pieces of myrrh were put in muslin bags and suspended on a cord between the breasts, where their fragrance would be released day and night by the warmth of the body.

Queen Hatshepsut wore a perfume containing the most highly prized fragrance of the East. Myrrh, a gum resin, is found in Yemen and southern Arabia and was widely used in perfumery as an ingredient of incense. The method of collecting this sticky substance has hardly changed at all over thousands of years. It is picked off the beards of goats which have fed on the shrub that it comes from. It is used today in the production of soap and shampoo. When mixed with wine or alcohol it has a narcotic effect, and during the Roman occupation of Palestine it is said to have been offered to prisoners on their way to crucifixion in order to numb their senses. Myrrh was associated with the goddess of the moon. Its main ingredients (like that of frankincense) have a similar chemical structure to human steroids, the male and female hormones, and it is possible that both may have an aphrodisiac effect.

Gums and resins such as myrrh continue to be added to ointments not only for their scent, but to 'fix' the fragrance of other ingredients. They are sometimes used in pot pourri today and are still burned in the home as incense.

PERFUMING AND DRESSING THE HAIR

One day an Iranian friend sat me down and announced that she was going to create a new hairstyle for a performance I was due to give that weekend. First she swept my hair onto the top of my head; then she took a brightly patterned scarf, folded it several times to create thickness and tied it across my forehead so that it framed my face. To this bandana she attached an old silver necklace and around this 'frontispiece' she looped several thin plaits (made from strands of my curly hair). Framing the face with colour and jewels sets it off in a very interesting way and the effect of this relatively simple headdress was dazzling. When we are not accustomed to taking this kind of trouble with our hair, it is a revelation to discover what effects can be obtained with relatively little time and assistance. For many of us, if our hair is looking good, we instantly feel confident; yet many women are wary of 'artificial' hair adornment. For some, perming and colouring is acceptable, but false hair of any kind is considered as 'beyond the pale' as false breasts.

In the East and in Africa women add false hair to their own hair as a matter of course. The nineteenth-century Ouled Nail women of Algeria were as famous for their elaborate headdresses as for their dancing. They wore high turbans and augmented their thick hair with plaits of oiled black sheep's wool wound round their ears. From a distance and on stage, this effect is perfectly splendid. A love of excess, of loading the hair and body with bright colours, the gleam of gold and silver all over the body, is inherent in women from African and Arab cultures. During the orientalist era it inspired a fashion among Europe's wealthy elite, and many a portrait of society women shows them decked out in oriental regalia, crowned by a jewelled turban. They threw parties where guests came in full oriental costume, and there was even a fashion for voluminous harem trousers. Early twentieth-century editions of *Vogue* magazine refer to *almeh*'s trousers, supposedly named (but in fact misnamed, for *almehs* were singers) after the newly popular dancers of the Arab world.

In North Africa a false piece is sometimes attached beneath a woman's real hair at the nape of the neck to give greater thickness; then the hair is arranged in loops on either side of the face. Depending on the thickness of this false piece, it is possible to create either a delicate or a theatrical effect.

In pharaonic frescos we find pictures showing women with cones of scented wax on their hair. When it grew warm, the fragrant wax melted down into the hair. This custom survived into the early twentieth century among certain bedouin tribes who lived in the desert in Egypt.

In parts of the Middle East, women still wear scented balls hidden in their long hair. In Saudi Arabia they perfume their hair with the smoke of incense when it is still wet after washing. After roughly towelling dry, a woman will hold her head over the incense burner so that the perfumed fumes rise and are trapped in her long hair, where the scent will linger for many hours afterwards. In the south-west of Saudi Arabia, in a valley surrounded by mountains, lies the city of Abha. Because of the difficulty of access, the culture of Abha had remained largely unchanged until recent times. It is a place where flowers grow abundantly, and in particular, the wonderful *full*, which has an intoxicating perfume. For celebrations, the women of Abha wear *full* headdresses like fitted caps over their hair, as well as plaits of glowing creamy-coloured flowers in their dark hair.

In many hot countries women weave flowers in their hair; sometimes it is a single red bloom, as in Spain and South America, and sometimes it is a rope of blossom woven into thin braids covering the entire head. In some countries a cluster of flowers is fixed at the base of a single long, thick braid.

Arranging the hair in countless thin plaits or braids is a long-established custom in North and black Africa and in the Middle East. Lady Mary Wortley Montagu, writing in the eighteenth century, described a Turkish woman with a small velvet cap perched on one side of the head and on the other a profusion of jewels of every description, together with highly scented flowers. 'It is hard to imagine anything more beautiful,' she concluded. In the East women loaded their bodies with jewellery; the arms were laden with bracelets, the ankles with bells or silver containers of dried beans, necklaces and amulets, all of which gave a gay glitter and tinkling as the women rustled about; scarves bordered with tiny coins also contributed to the festive percussion which announced a woman's arrival. Lady Mary noted that when women braided their hair, the braids were always of an odd number because even numbers were considered unlucky (hence *The Thousand and One Nights*):

> Into each of these braids, or thin plaited tresses of hair, three strings of black silk, some eighteen inches in length, are woven, to which an immense number of small gold spangles are fastened at irregular intervals. Sometimes the silken threads, which are called keytans, are attached to a lace or band of black silk which is bound round the head, and they then hang quite separately from the plaits of hair. The spangles are flat, thin ornaments of gold, all of the same size and shape, called 'bark', and there are about twelve bark to each string. By a tiny ring at their upper extremities these sequin-like spangles are fastened to the silken strings, an inch apart, but those of each string are carefully arranged so as not to correspond with those of the other strings. At the end of each of the strings is a small gold tube (masoorah), or else a many-sided gold bead (habbeh), and beneath this is suspended by a tiny ring a gold coin about five eighths of an inch in diameter. Other forms of ending to the strings are occasionally used by rich women in place of gold coins. One of these is a flat ornament composed of open filigree gold work with a pearl in the centre, whilst at times a tiny tassle of pearls ends the keytan, or string. Sometimes each keytan ends alternately with a pearl and an emerald. The countless gold spangles almost entirely hide the hair, and glitter and tinkle with every movement of the head.

Turbans

A turban is a protective device against the heat of the sun. If you are visiting a hot country, packing a couple of long scarves or a sarong to make into a turban is more useful than taking along a sunhat, for it can also double as a beach wrap (or cover an ugly table or lampshade).

You can make a simple turban to keep off the sun by winding a single length of fabric around the head, Indian style. Position the end of the fabric on the crown of the head so that it is draped over the back to the nape of the neck. Keep one hand on the crown to secure the material and with the other hand begin winding it horizontally around the head. When you have finished, tuck the end tightly underneath.

For a more decorative party turban, take several lengths of material or scarves in contrasting colours. Use the first scarf to cover the hair, tying it at the nape of the neck.

Over this arrange four or five scarves or strips of fabric of contrasting colour and weight – glittering, patterned, plain, whatever comes to hand. Fold them and twist them to create texture and thickness and wind them round your head. Fix them in place by simply tucking them in at the ends. You shouldn't need to use clips. The final scarf can be twisted into a sausage, with a string of pearls or a silver necklace woven into it before it is firmly secured.

As a final touch you may like to arrange a coin necklace in a loop across your forehead, tucking the ends into your turban or else securing it more firmly with hair grips. You can also secure it by using a length of thin elastic passing under the hair at the nape of the neck.

Threading Pearls in the Hair

For her wedding, my Iranian friend strung rows of symmetrical pearls in her lustrous black hair. When she moved her head they swung delicately to and fro, seemingly suspended magically in her hair, for they were so artfully woven in that even if you looked closely it was impossible to discover how they were secured!

This wonderful effect can be created just as well on short hair as on long, but like all the best decorative effects, it takes time. Here is how it is done:

Apart from the decorations you intend using, you will need a small size of lead-free shot (the kind that fisherman use) and a small pair of plyers. Every sequin, bead or pearl is attached by threading it onto a single strand of hair (unless you have perfect vision you will have to invest in a needle-threader for this part of the operation!).

Thread a single item of decoration onto a strand of hair. Add a piece of shot directly beneath the decoration, and close with the plyers, which will keep both items in place. The shot is essential to prevent the decorating from falling off. In this way you can arrange spangles and jewels, either in symmetrical lines or scattered randomly in the hair. Sequins are easy to use because they are light, while the shot is obviously heavier.

Afro-Caribbean Plaiting

The curly structure of African hair allows moisture to escape more easily than Caucasian hair, and consequently makes it more dry and brittle but too much washing can remove essential hair oils. This kind of hair needs frequent oiling to keep it in good condition, and one of the reasons why braiding is so popular is that it stops the hair drying out. It also helps the hair grow thick and long.

Plaiting or braiding the hair can take a couple of hours or more, but the braids can be left in for several weeks. Washing the hair is then a simple matter of running streams of water through the braids, which tend to pick up less dirt than hair which is left hanging loose. (However, pulling the hair very tightly into braids tends to weaken and even break it, so it's not advisable to maintain this style all the time.) If you have braids you can also massage henna wax into your hair; you can then wrap it in a hot towel and let the wax do its work while you relax in the bath.

There are numerous styles of Afro-Caribbean braiding. It is the custom for hair to be partly braided during childhood; then after puberty the styles become increasingly complex.

Braids can be left hanging loose, they can be wound round the head or they can be secured in a bun at the nape of the neck. A lovely effect can be created by weaving gold or silver thread into the braids. Flowers, sequins, shells and beads can all be woven in, and I have seen some stunning effects, using this method of decorating the hair.

CORNROWING. This is the most common form of braiding. Comb the hair to straighten out any tight, kinky curls. Make a centre parting from the front of the hairline to the nape of the neck. Secure half the parted hair with a comb or clips. Divide the other half into three equal, longitudinal sections.

Starting with the section furthest from the top of the head and working from back to front, take three small portions of hair and braid them firmly into a three-fold strand which lies flat on the scalp. Continue in this way by picking up hair from the roots at short intervals and weaving it into each strand. At the front, braid the hair to the very top and twist the ends for a tidy finish.

Repeat this process on the other two sections of hair, making your way to the top of the head. Repeat the cornrowing with the other half of your hair.

You should oil your scalp every day to avoid dandruff. Coconut oil, palm oil and shea butter are all popularly used in the Caribbean.

CROSS-BRAIDING. Cross-braiding involves cornrowing one braid over another, which has the effect of giving the style more height.

WEAVING. Weaving is cornrowing using an attachment or hair extensions. They are first attached and then the cornrowing is done; the ends of the braids are stitched together using a needle and thread. The ends are then rolled up and stitched into position.

THREADING. Threading is a technique of wrapping sectioned hair with thread. You will need a wooden Afro comb, hair oil, a pair of scissors or a razor blade and spools of thread. To guard against scalp tension, wrap the hair evenly and avoid pulling it by wrapping it too tightly.

Comb the hair to get rid of knots. Divide it into sixteen sections and secure each one with clips or rubber bands, leaving out only the one which you are working on.

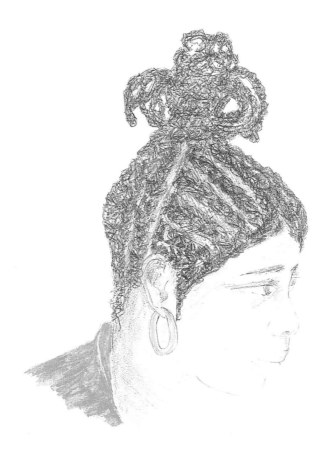

Oil the section which you are about to thread. Take 1 m (3 ft) of doubled-up thread in your right hand and hold the oiled section of hair firmly at the scalp between your left thumb and forefinger. Having anchored the end of the thread by twisting it round the hair at the scalp, wind the thread clockwise around the section, moving gradually towards the ends of the hair. When you arrive at the very tip, knot the thread securely two or three times so that it does not unravel. Cut off the end of the thread.

Repeat this process with each of the other sections until all the hair has been threaded. Oil the scalp every day.

This style can be left in for about a week, but it should be unwrapped and washed after that. It encourages the hair to grow faster but constant threading may make the hairline recede from the temples, so it is advisable to alternate this style with cornrowing.

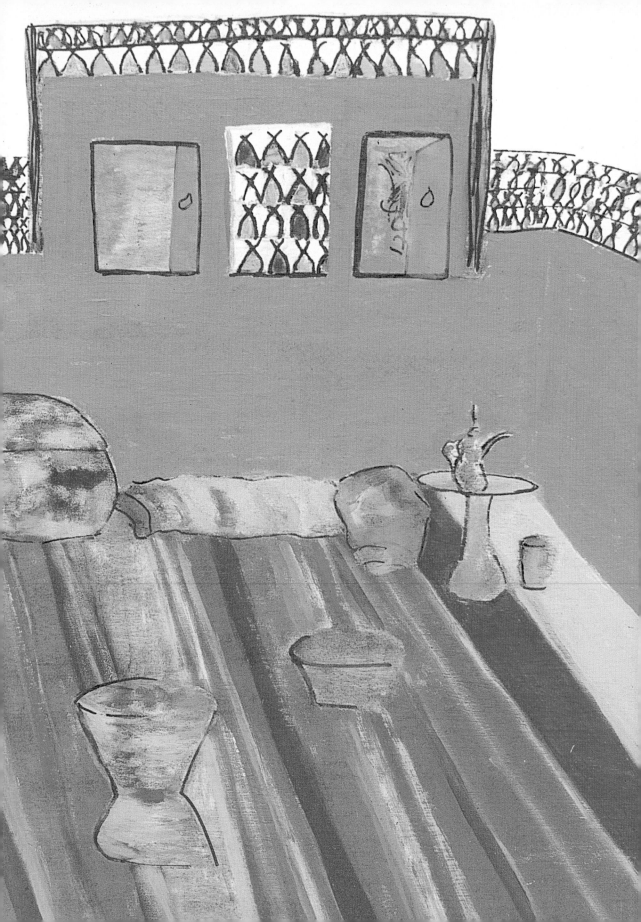

7
Ambience and Celebration

As she withdrew, the lissom maid,
This way and that she gently swayed
As a narcissus 'neath the trees
Swings on its stem before the breeze.

Deep in his heart the lover hears
The pendants hanging from her ears
Ring out a tender melody:
'I love thee dearly: lov'st thou me?'

(Ibn Hazm, *The Ring of the Dove*)

I remember talking once to an Iranian woman who had spent her youth moving from country to country with her diplomat father. Although they did not take all their furniture with them on their travels, they always took along a trunkload of beautiful carpets. She remembers once, lying in bed ill and in low spirits, wondering if she was ever going to get better, when her father opened the door and came into the room bearing a carpet. He then brought in a series of rugs one by one and arranged them round the room for her to look at. 'I lay there gazing at the patterns and colours and they were so beautiful I went into a kind of meditation,' she said. 'I could feel my spirits lift and after a while I started to feel better.'

In a world where there is so much to distress us, we cannot overestimate the effect of beauty on our state of mind.

The words 'Feast your eyes' with which carpet merchants usher you into their shops seem to me to describe perfectly the effect of looking at oriental rugs, which cover the floor with jewel-like splendour. They are truly a feast for the eyes and I am always perturbed in carpet shops to see tourists tramping around in their outdoor shoes, treading the dirt and grime of the streets into what are essentially exquisite works of art.

Unfortunately, we have never developed a tradition in the West of removing our shoes when we go indoors; but it is a widespread ritual in the East to do so. On the porches of Indian and South-East Asian homes you will always find a row of abandoned shoes kicked off by their owners as they step inside. The Japanese have a pair of slippers for every room in the house, including ones with w.c. printed on them for wearing in the toilet.

Removing outdoor shoes is one of those customs which indicate the scrupulous care placed on cleanliness in many countries of the East. There are other rituals of cleanliness, considered vital in terms of both creating a pleasurable home environment and welcoming visitors to one's home.

In Islam hospitality and generosity to strangers are central tenets of life. It is a duty which is taken seriously, and it is often those who can least afford it who are the most generous in inviting a stranger to sit down and share their food and drink. To persuade a visitor to stay and dine in one's house is a kind of triumph and at the same time an honour for the host. In the words of an old Arab saying: 'If a stranger is standing at your door, do not shut it in their face.' Hospitality is considered a duty to friends and strangers alike. For the desert bedouin of the past, eking out an existence in the harshest of surroundings, to turn away strangers from one's tent was perhaps to condemn them to death; for the next well, the next drinkable water, might have been many kilometres away.

The dream of those who live in arid places is of water and greenery. To desert dwellers they are the stuff of poetry. In his book *What Am I Doing Here?* Bruce Chatwin tells the story of a shanty town in Marseilles where Algerian guest workers lived. He noticed in one makeshift hut that the sole decoration pinned on the wall by the young boy who lived there was a picture of two gladioli which he had torn out of a bulb merchant's catalogue.

In Andalusia, Arabs and Berbers (known as Moors) ruled for nearly 500 years and left their mark in the fountains and flowered courtyards attached to houses. In the rest of Europe, at a time when the concept of having fresh running water in the home did not exist, the Moors of Andalusia had already established a comprehensive water distribution system which exists to this day.

Flowers and fragrance have a vital part to play in creating a soothing, welcoming atmosphere. In ancient Egypt the first duty towards guests was to perfume their wigs with scented oils, and in India and South-East Asia today garlands of flowers are still placed round the neck of a new arrival.

When perfume is diffused through a warm room, it prevents the free passage of heat rays and reduces the temperature. In India the roots of cuscus (vetiver) are incorporated into sun blinds. This root gives off a delicate violet scent when the blinds are watered, as is done throughout the day, to keep down the temperature.

In Palestine people used to place branches of fresh green leaves over the bed for their cooling properties. They also added dried herbs and flowers, selected for their soporific qualities, to the stuffing of mattresses and pillows.

Saudi Arabia is one of many countries where incense is burned at the entrance to the home in order to create a soothing atmosphere. Traditionally, guests are invited to hold their clothes over the incense to perfume them; after they have been seated and served with sweets and fruit, the incense burner is brought over so that they may perfume their hair with its fumes. At the end of the evening when it is time to leave, the incense is brought in again and passed round as a sign that the party is over. After this, it would be impolite for guests to linger beneath their host's roof. Incense burners are also placed in the wardrobe for a short while to perfume clothes.

In India and Iran incense is burned in front of a portrait of someone who has died, to help their soul rise to the next level of existence. In Iran rosewater is sprinkled over the family on their way to a funeral, to mitigate their sadness. In fact, there are few areas of human experience for which perfume has no role to play. Throughout India, the Gulf and Saudi Arabia, incense is used to alleviate depression. It is sprinkled over the heads of guests at weddings; it is burned in a room prior to going on a journey for luck and safety; and it is also thought to help dispel bad feelings from a room. It is certainly true that pleasant aromas work wonders on the subconscious; they can lift the spirits and put us in a new frame of mind.

One of the most popular substances used in incense is *bahour*, a form of frankincense. At weddings in Tunisia it is burned throughout the night. It is mixed with musk and pulverized ambergris and heated in a pan until it has acquired a jelly-like consistency. After it has been left to cool down, it is made into little balls which are stored in airtight jars. Finely wrought brass incense burners, for hanging and placing on the floor, are beautiful objects in themselves and using them creates long-lasting fragrance in the home. However, it is something of an art to keep these burners going. Like fires they need to be tended, topped up with extra charcoal and incense at regular intervals, and today people sometimes take the easy way out and use electric burners instead.

Using an Incense Burner

If you have a fire or stove already lit, take some glowing embers and place them in the bowl of the incense burner. If not, you will need to heat some lozenges of charcoal (which you can buy in a hardware shop) until they are red-hot. You will probably need to blow gently on them for a few minutes to get them going.

Now throw on the incense. If it comes from a block, crumble a little onto the coals. One of my favourites is benzoin (which, incidentally, is the main ingredient in Friar's Balsam). It comes in solid white pieces with glittering brown veins and leaves a rich, lingering fragrance behind it.

Other Ways of Using Fragrance in the Home

An easy method for creating fragrance in a room is to use a pottery fragrancer, which you can buy in health food and other similar shops. In the bottom there is a space for a night light, and in the top a bowl which can be filled with water and a few drops of your favourite essential oil.

Many of these oils have anti-bacterial properties, so apart from using them to scent a room they will also purify the air when someone is sick. Women who have given birth in rooms scented with essential oils have reported that the soothing, uplifting fragrance helped calm them and made the experience more bearable.

In the past certain illnesses were treated by burning scented oils; the Assyrians used fumigations of cannabis to lift depression and syphilis was treated with inhalations of burning cinnabar.

If you don't have a fragrancer simply add a few drops of oil to a bowl of warm water and place it near a radiator or fire; or soak a few drops in a cotton wool ball and tuck it by the radiator pipe.

You can also sprinkle 1 or 2 drops onto the light bulb in a table lamp, and as the bulb heats up it will give off a delicate fragrance. But remember that ESSENTIAL OILS ARE INFLAMMABLE, so you should only apply them to the light bulb when it is cold and the table lamp is switched off.

You can add 1 or 2 drops to the melted wax of a candle, but once again, remember that these oils are inflammable, so be careful not to get them on the wick.

If you have a wood fire burning in winter, add 1 drop of oil to each log half an hour before using. (The wood will retain the scent for a long time, so don't think you have to use any more than a drop for each log). Cypress, cedarwood, pine and sandalwood are ideal.

You can also sprinkle clean, dry towels or underwear with scent and put them on a radiator to warm before using them.

An Antiseptic Room Freshener

Add a few drops of bergamot or lavender to the water in a heated room fragrancer. Or add to a bowl of water and place on a radiator or other source of heat. Other antiseptic oils which smell pleasing as a room freshener include pine, geranium, basil, cinnamon and clove.

For those who have the time, here are some household fragrancers to make:

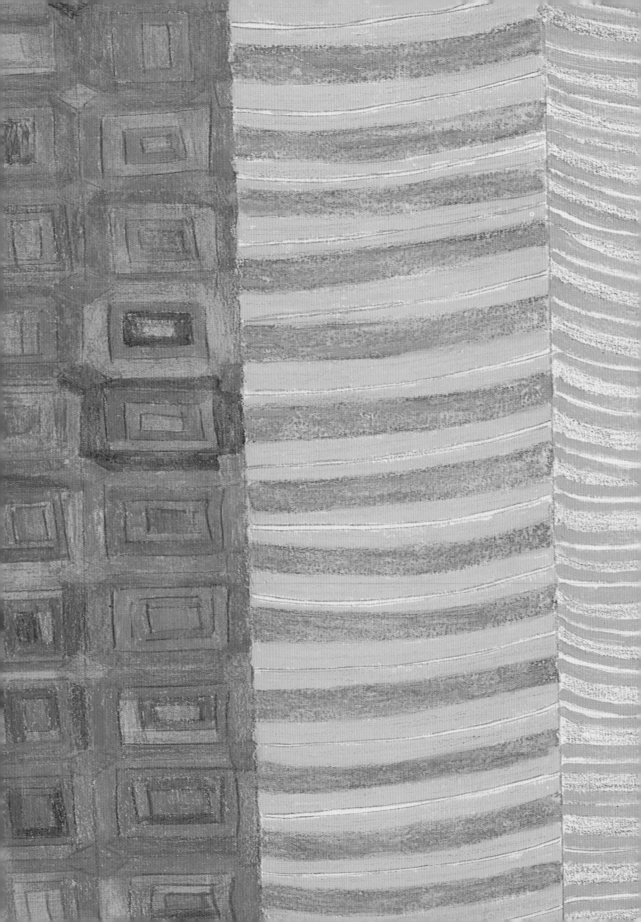

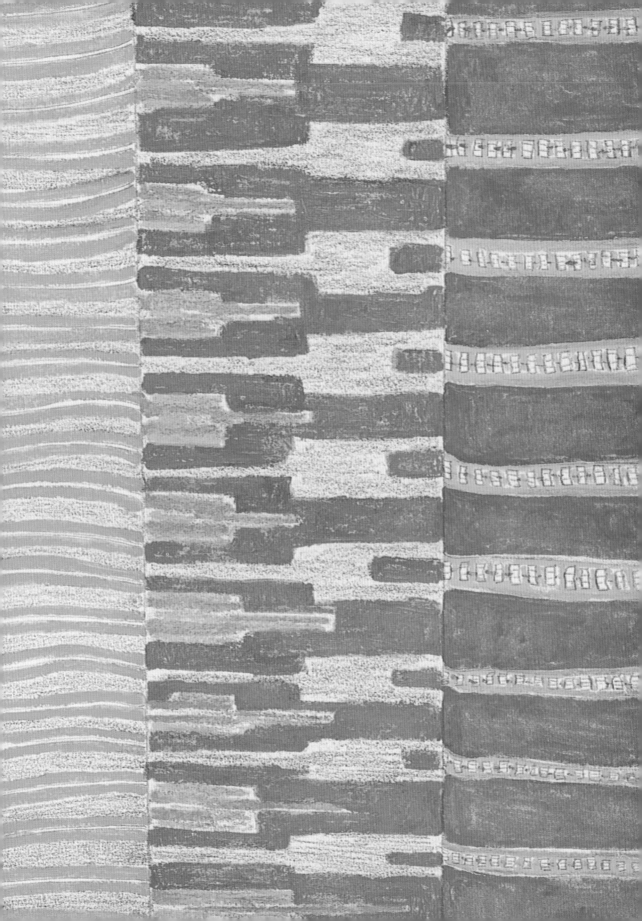

Spice Balls

Spice balls can be made with any combination of pot pourri ingredients – flowers, seeds, gums and leaves – pounded together in a pestle and mortar. Add a sufficient amount of gum tragacanth and rosewater to make a sticky, dough-like paste. Roll this dough into little balls and leave them to dry in the air. Store them in a box or jar (not a plastic bag, which will keep them soft and eventually encourage a mould to form on them).

A suggested combination of fragrances:

90 g (3 oz) powdered orris root

30 g (1 oz) cassia

30 g (1 oz) lavender flowers

30 g (1 oz) cloves

15 g (½ oz) rhodium wood

1 teaspoon vanilla

15–20 drops oil of verbena

½ cup of rosewater or a few drops of rose essence.

Optional extras: a few drops of musk, ambergris or tincture of benzoin.

Fragrance Pillows

For sweet dreams, mix well-dried rose petals with sweet basil, dried mint and pounded cloves and stuff a small pillow with this mixture.

THE EROTIC ARTS

A humid kiss is better than a hurried coitus.

(Sheikh Nefzawi, *The Perfumed Garden*)

The first time Cleopatra invited Antony to dine with her she ordered the floors to be strewn knee-deep in rose petals. The Egyptian queen was worshipped as Isis, the goddess of love. Her favourite perfume contained the scent of crocus, rose and violet; she anointed her feet with aegyptium, an almond-oil lotion containing cinnamon, honey, orange blossom and henna, and used a different fragrance for each part of her body. Roses were suspended in nets on the walls of her palace and even the sails of her barge were drenched with perfume.

The language and lore of sensuality in the ancient literature of the East makes intoxicating reading. Stories of erotic encounters describe the orchestration of sight, sound, touch, taste and smell as being vital to a fulfilling sexual rendezvous, with many suggestions for creating a sensual ambience:

> Tomorrow morning, erect a tent of many coloured silks. Spread rich silken fabric on the ground. Sprinkle it with perfumes of rose petal, orange flower, eglantine, jasmine, carnation, violet and other essences. Then in golden containers burn incense. Take care to make the tent airtight so that none of the scents may escape. When the smoke of the incense has mingled with the odours of the scented waters, take your place upon your throne and wait for her. Then receive her in the tent alone. When she has smelt so many odours, everything within her will soften. She will become intoxicated. She will almost lose consciousness. Then make advances to her worthy of a man such as yourself . . .
>
> (Sheikh Nefzawi, *The Perfumed Garden*)

Anointing the room with fragrance to satisfy the sense of smell was only one of many suggestions for creating an all-embracing atmosphere of sensual delight; aside from this, there was adorning the body to stimulate the sight; listening to music and poetry to soothe the ears; and partaking of food and drink containing aphrodisiac ingredients to awaken the tastebuds and rouse the libido.

Many types of food have, in their time, been claimed to have an aphrodisiac effect, and it is true that certain spices do stimulate the nervous system more than others. One of these is nutmeg, which contains a type of hallucinogenic amphetamine, as well as being highly poisonous when taken in large quantities. Cooked celery contains a substance akin to the chemical pheromones secreted by insects, humans and other animals as a method of mutual attraction. Basil, cinnamon, cloves, ginger and asparagus are all on the list of foods with supposedly aphrodisiac qualities. (However, according to modern science, the connection we often make between food and sex is simply down to the fact that the inside of the mouth and the sex organs in our species share a similar type of nerve ending.) But who needs to consult an expert to know that eating a meal in beguiling surroundings with someone attractive is psychically seductive, whether or not a certain food is on the menu?

However, there are some aphrodisiacs (with a long history of use in the East) which contain poisons that not only cause severe stomach and liver disorders, but can ultimately prove fatal. Among them is Cantarides, the notorious 'Spanish fly', which comes from the wings of a species of beetle. It was used as a sexual stimulant in North Africa and throughout the Mediterranean and, more prosaically, to burn off warts. Several hours after applying it externally to the body the skin would start to blister, so we can imagine what it must have done to the stomach. In fact, this highly toxic substance works by irritating the genito-urinary tract. The Marquis de Sade used it as a filling for chocolates (in his day chocolate

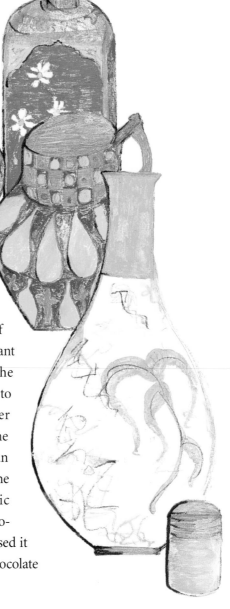

often contained opium, a well-known sensual enhancer) and it is also mentioned as a cooking ingredient in old Moroccan cookery books. You can still find Spanish fly in the spice souks of North Africa and the Middle East, as well as other dubious-sounding aphrodisiacs such as 'Dragon's tail' and 'Ogre's milk' – survivals of a trade in love philtres promising that most highly sought-after human experience: sexual satisfaction.

There are several intriguing recipes for aphrodisiacs in the secular literature of the East; some are to be eaten and others are to be massaged into the skin or inserted in various bodily orifices. Women are advised to mix the powdered stems of lavender and rosemary and insert them in the vagina so that they give off a delicate scent. If you don't fancy this, then substituting little silver balls is recommended for increasing one's pleasure by providing a rhythmic, melodic accompaniment to love-making.

Kissing is treated at length in *The Perfumed Garden*, which gives examples of appropriate and inappropriate types of kisses. Be warned then that: 'The kiss given to the superficial outer part of the lips, and making a noise comparable to the one by which you call your cat, gives no pleasure.'

A woman who is less than enthusiastic about love-making is advised to mix powdered camomile and asphodel in lubin oil and smear it all over her vagina. This will apparently make her burn with desire so that she will not rest until she is satisfied.

But more useful by far than any of these suggestions is, I think, Sheikh Nefzawi's advice to men:

> A woman is like basil; if one wishes to savour its perfume, one must take its leaves between one's fingers and rub them; then the plant will give off its scent. Otherwise one will get nothing, for it will jealously keep its delectable essence.

THE GARDENS OF PARADISE

The word paradise comes from the Persian *pairi* ('around') and *daeza* ('wall'); thus we discover that the ideal Islamic retreat is an enclosed garden, a place of beautiful yet contained nature. The earliest Persian gardens, dating back to 2000 BC, were known as *chahar bagh*, or fourfold gardens. Islamic gardens are similarly designed: square or rectangular enclosures divided into four parts, leading to a life-giving spring in the middle. Geometry and symmetry are of prime importance, with the four divisions marked out by channels of water meeting in a central pool or fountain. Water is vital to the Islamic garden, the greatest value being placed on this natural source of life, so scarce in the arid climate of the Middle East. Paradise is a place overflowing with water, and in Islamic gardens all containers are kept topped up with this most precious of fluids. The sound of running water, tinkling in fountains and splashing over stones, adds a harmonious sound to the tranquillity of the Islamic garden, which is designed as a sanctuary, a place to soothe and calm the spirits. The Persians used to float hundreds of tiny candles on the pools at night, whose light, reflected in the water, must have been a magical sight. Plants for the Islamic garden were carefully chosen for their scent, with citrus smells predominant.

In a similar vein, the paradise of the Qur'an is a retreat, a place of sublime beauty and sensual delight. It is a land of the most intense pleasures imaginable, where each of the five senses is perpetually feasted beyond any point that is remotely conceivable. Nature is eternally in bloom, and such nature as we have never seen before. One type of tree is described as having a trunk covered in pearl and filled with fragrant hyacinths; it has branches made of glittering topaz and leaves of spun silk. Hyacinths and gold, emeralds and sapphires, coral and diamonds are the fabric of this artificial heaven where we may eat and drink to our heart's content without the inconvenience of digestion. When we enter paradise, our breath becomes scented with musk; every day we grow more beautiful and our appetite increases. Most important of all, our erotic satisfaction is not only assured, it is infinitely greater than anything we could ever contemplate on earth. In the desert the thirst is never quenched, but the musk-scented waters of paradise will quench our thirst forever.

However, despite a passing mention of female desire, this is a paradise geared strictly to the satisfaction of the male sex. It is staffed by female slaves who do the menial work and houris whose *raison d'être* is the satisfaction of male desire. As soon as a man enters paradise he is given seventy of these houris, and if he has observed the fast of Ramadan he is awarded a special black-eyed houri who lives in a tent made of white pearl. We should not be surprised to discover that there is no male equivalent of the houri to cater to female desire. Houris have their husband's name branded on their breast; they are creatures 'as feminine as can be imagined . . . from the toes to the knees they are made of saffron, from the knees to the breast of musk, from the breast to the neck of amber, from the neck to the top of their heads of camphor'. In paradise a man's sexual prowess is heightened so that 'each climax is extended and extended and lasts for twenty-four years'. It is scarcely to be wondered that men are eager to sacrifice themselves in holy wars on earth when they are assured of immediate transportation to this extraordinary land of erotic surfeit.

> Glory to Allah, who did not create
> A more enchanting spectacle than that of two happy lovers;
> Drunk with voluptuous delights
> They lie on their couch,
> Their arms entwined,
> Their hands clasped,
> Their hearts beating in tune.
> (*The Thousand and One Nights*)

It is instructive to contrast the attitudes of different world faiths on the subject of eroticism. In Indian Tantra, the object of sexuality is to attain a higher plane of consciousness and union with the divine. A woman anoints her body with different fragrances to arouse the different senses: jasmine for the hands, patchouli for the cheeks and neck, spikenard for the hair, amber for the nipples, saffron for the feet, sandalwood for the inner thighs and musk for the pubis.

Christianity, as we might expect, has never had much truck with sensual pleasures. St Paul warned men against having anything to do with women, citing celibacy as the human ideal, and it is fortunate that at least some people didn't take his ideas seriously.

As for Judaism, it consistently thunders against sensual pleasure. In the Book of Proverbs, men are cautioned against a woman who perfumes her bed with myrrh, aloes and cinnamon and told to avoid women whose glinting and tinkling jewellery announces their presence. Yet the Old Testament also contains something quite extraordinary – The Song of Songs, which celebrates human beauty and the joys of sexuality:

> Thou hast ravished my heart with one of thine eyes,
> With one chain of thy neck.
> How fair is thy love,
> How much better is thy love than wine!
> And the smell of thine ointments than all the spices!
> Thy lips, O my beloved, drop as the honeycomb;
> Honey and milk are under thy tongue;
> And the smell of thy garments is like the smell of Lebanon.
> A garden enclosed is my beloved;
> A spring shut up, a fountain sealed.
> Thy plants are an orchard of pomegranates with pleasant fruits;
> Camphire, with spikenard,
> Spikenard and saffron;
> Calamus and cinnamon, with all trees of frankincense;
> Myrrh and aloes, with all the spices . . .
> Set me as a seal upon thine heart, as a seal upon thine arm:
> For love is strong as death.

The Song of Songs is an enigma. There we find it, in the middle of a book devoted to homilies on moral righteousness, flanked by the thundering of a jealous, vengeful God exhorting his people to wage war on their enemies. Discovering page upon page of a beautiful love song in this context is like seeing a gorgeous butterfly living in a nest of hornets, and we shall never know the mystery of quite how it came to be there.

PERSIAN NEW YEAR (*NOROUZ*)

Thirteen days after the Persian New Year, if you happen to be in central London, you will be treated to the sight of Iranian families carrying little pots of green shoots, walking through Hyde Park towards the Serpentine. There, as the final part of their celebrations, they will throw their pots into the waters which snake through the middle of the park.

Persian New Year falls on 21 March, the first day of spring, and is marked by extravagant festivities. On the table is placed a *haft seen*, which consists of at least seven items beginning with the letter 's'. In pre-Islamic times the table was set with a *haft sheen* (seven items beginning with 'sh'). These included *shokafa* (blossoms), *shireeni* (sweets), *sham* (candles), *shekair* (sugar) and *sheer* (milk). However, wine (*sharab*) was also included, and as alcohol is forbidden to Muslims, the 'sh' was later replaced by an 's'; the wine was removed from the table and replaced by vinegar (*serke*).

Today's *haft seen* could include *seeb* (apple), *seer* (garlic), *sombol* (hyacinths), *sekea* (coins), *somagh* (a dried herb), *senjet* (dried berries) and *samanoo* (a sweet desert, made only for New Year celebrations). Also part of the *haft seen* is a mirror to represent light, goldfish to bring health and prosperity, and a pot of *sabse* (green shoots) to symbolize a plentiful harvest. In addition there is a copy of the Qur'an, within whose pages are placed fresh new banknotes to be given to children.

The *haft seen* is left for thirteen days, and then the green shoots are taken out and thrown in a river or running water. On this day, too, it is the tradition to go for a picnic; an Iranian friend laughingly told me that this is the day when most burglaries occur because everyone is out picnicking and taking their pots of shoots to throw in the water!

MARRIAGE RITES

I am He, says man to woman in front of the fire witness,
You are She.
I am the melody,
You are the words.
I am the sky,
You are the earth.
Let us now be one.
From us let children spring.
(Indian wedding recitation)

Many years ago I was invited to a village wedding in the south of Morocco. My memory of it is compounded of flavours and scents: the full-blown scent of night-blooming jasmine, entering at the open window; the sharp tang of lemon essence sprinkled onto my hands as we all sat down to eat; the aromatic steam rising from the chicken *tagine* (stew), laden with saffron and cumin and coriander. And then later the sensation of warm honey dripping down my arm as I helped myself to cakes fresh from the oven.

I had met the bridegroom, a young boy who ran a jewellery stall in the souk, a day earlier. After chatting for ten minutes he invited my partner and me to his wedding and was most insistent that we come.

Which of us in the West would think of inviting a perfect stranger to our wedding? Which of us would sit them down at the dinner table and offer them the best of everything, before even our closest friends and family had eaten? But there are many countries where this scenario is regarded as perfectly normal.

Having a stranger at the feast is considered lucky; it's benign magic, and at the same time it fulfils the obligation to share one's good fortune.

Part of the wedding rituals in many Asian and Middle Eastern countries involves a street procession, accompanied by music, singing and dancing, and it is not unusual for passers-by to find themselves caught up in these festivities or observing from the sidelines.

A riot of bright colours and copious quantities of flowers are also essential to wedding celebrations. In India shades of red and orange are the favourite colours and you will never see a bride wearing white, which is the Indian colour of death and mourning.

In the dirt and pollution of Delhi's city streets one is suddenly brought up short by the sight of heaps of flowers, dazzling gold and orange and yellow, piled on the ground. Men sit cross-legged around these mounds of gorgeous blossoms, still wet with dew, threading flower chains, many basketloads of which are used in a wedding ceremony.

An Indian bride has her entire body bathed in bright yellow turmeric paste, which leaves her skin silky soft and several shades lighter in tone. Her hair is washed with 'three fruits', dried over incense, then oiled and arranged in coils to frame her face. Her make-up is more elaborate than usual, with gold and silver dots painted all round the eye socket, and gold glitter rubbed all over her body. The marriage bed is covered with the finest silks, each one a classic of its kind, and boxes of ancestral jewels are opened up for her to choose from. She will wear these jewels on her wedding night for the first and only time, and after that they will be put away and stored for her own children in the years to come.

In other countries besides India (and depending on a family's wealth), wedding festivities may go on for several days, with each day allotted its special ritual. For the bride the most important one is the day spent at the baths, a day of cleansing, beauty treatments and the ritual adornment of the hair and body with henna. It is the last of many cleansing and beautifying rituals which precede her wedding night and is an occasion of much merriment among the women. The application of henna is always an excuse for a party, for it requires several hours to take effect. If they can afford it, the family engages the services of a professional henna painter; if not, then friends and family take on the task instead. A skilled henna painter who can create intricate designs is much in demand. It is a good profession for a young woman, for it enables her to move around freely in public in the exercise of her craft. In strict Muslim countries where women are not encouraged to take a public role, henna painting is among the most socially respected methods of earning a living.

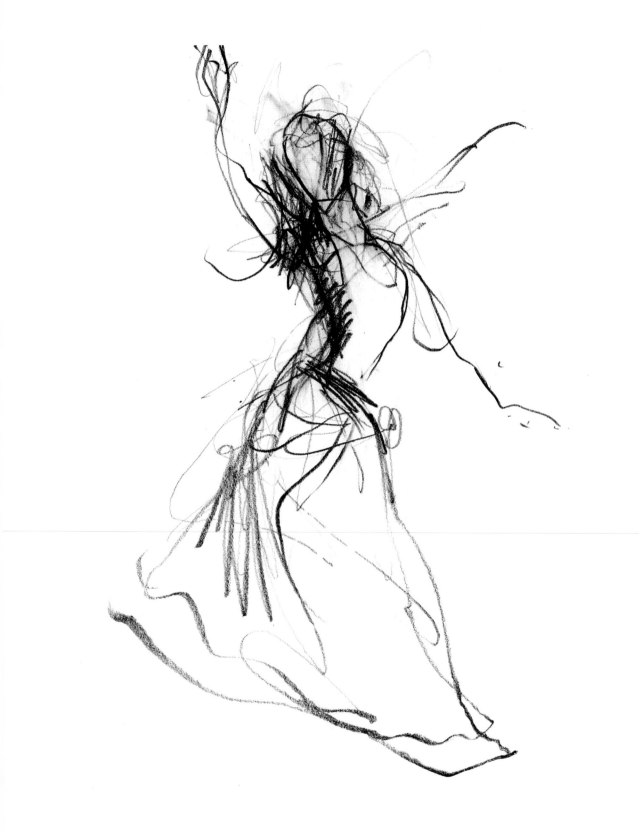

DANCE

Those slimly dancing bodies sway
Like the swaying of green reeds,
Or as the grasses wave.
Glances shoot from the eyes,
Like long brown arrows dipped in gold.

('Ten Young Girls in a Meadow', *The Thousand and One Nights*)

An Iranian friend recently took me to a women's party in London. Her friends were in their forties and fifties, and were elegantly dressed as for a night out on the town (indeed, one of them changed into a second splendid outfit halfway through the evening when she wanted to entertain the rest of us with a special dance!). They had sent the men away so that they could let down their hair and enjoy themselves without any disapproving glances.

'If they start dancing *ruhozy*,' my friend said, 'one of the men is sure to object – especially if it's his wife and there are other men present. So we get rid of the men first!'

Persian *ruhozy*-dancing is bawdy and comical and a lot of fun. The women at the party, who had lived in exile for many years, had spent their lives jet-setting round the capitals of the world. Yet when they really wanted to enjoy themselves they kicked off their shoes and had fun in the traditional way, getting up one by one to dance while the others clapped or sang along with the music. They were still going strong in the early hours of the morning, and the only time a shadow passed over the merriment was when they fell into a reverie, listening to old Persian music which reminded them of all they had lost in leaving the land of their birth.

In many cultures, from earliest times down to the present day, dancers have been thought to bring good fortune, especially at weddings. No celebration is complete without their presence, though in the Arab-Islamic world the professional dancer has an ambiguous status for complex reasons. Yet dancing in private is another matter. Little girls grow up learning to imitate their mothers at informal parties, dancing by moving their hips and arms in subtle, lyrical and playful ways. In Egypt, dancing in private among women is still a means whereby a young girl can advertise her charms in front of a prospective mother-in-law!

The most enjoyable parties are often informal ones, occasions when people suddenly find themselves together and dance and music arise spontaneously out of the spirit of the moment. The Tunisian performer Leyla Haddad described impromptu family parties back home in Djerba: 'My uncle is a wonderful *oud* (lute) player. It isn't his profession, but he has played for many years. Sometimes in the evening, out of the blue, if he feels like it, he picks up his *oud*. And he can play for hours and hours. The neighbours come in, one person brings another, and so from five people we become twenty-five! And those who can sing, they sing, and then people start getting up to dance and so, out of nothing, there is a feast! Because, all of a sudden, the mood is here, the people are here, one song leads to another, and it becomes a magic night.'

In recent years Western women have fallen under the spell of Arabic dance, which now has an enormous following. One of them commented to me: 'When I first saw an Egyptian dancer my jaw dropped. I realized I was sitting there and my mouth had fallen open! I just thought, Oh, I want my body to move like that. It was so beautiful.' When I too first saw Arabic dance it spoke to me personally, and over many years of teaching it I have seen thousands of women become similarly inspired by it.

All dance is about sensual expression. It is about energy and vitality, and it is one of the most liberating activities available to us. As a way of letting off steam, socializing and expressing ourselves it has no rival. When we step onto the dance floor we leave our worries at the door. When we're feeling flat, dance recharges our battery; and if we're under the weather, by the end of an evening of dance the chances are we will be feeling fine again.

Dancing releases a chemical in the body which promotes well-being, and when this is sustained over a period of hours (as in trance dancing) it can lead to a state of ecstasy without recourse to alcohol or other drugs. But of course, no one dances because they think it's going to do them good, though they may go to exercise classes for just that reason.

But there is no natural place for physical activity of a vigorous, creative and expressive nature in our increasingly sedentary lives. As a doctor friend of mine confessed: 'A group of us were sitting talking the other day and we all came to the conclusion that what was missing in our lives was dancing.'

Many people have begun going to dance classes because they recognize, however subconsciously, that they have a physical energy which needs to be discharged. Multicultural dance forms such as flamenco, tango, African and Arabic dance have all attracted a huge following in recent years, and I think this is partly because all these forms share a challenging and passionate sensuality. Different dance forms have different things to offer, and we each find the one which satisfies our own particular needs.

Unlike Western dance which, broadly speaking, uses a large space and is based on movement of the limbs, both Arabic and African dance centre on an articulated torso. The energy in this underused part of the body is brought back to life and reunited with the rest of the body so that it flows without being blocked or checked. Both dance forms are earthy and strongly rooted, and are based on a wealth of movement in the pelvis, seat not only of intense sensation but of our deepest taboos. Exploring movement in this part of the body can be a source of liberation for many women, and in the case of Arabic dance, the shimmering, serpentine hip and torso movements are a great attraction.

Mastering a new dance – especially one from an unfamiliar culture – involves a lot of sweat. It also involves the control of muscles and an appreciation of music (it may be a completely unfamiliar kind of music) and in the process it introduces us to a different culture, even a different way of life. Learning any dance form, we are forced to take a good look at what kind of self-image we have and how we present ourselves to the world. Dance is an acute barometer of self-esteem. When we dance we reveal, through our posture and the ease or difficulty with which we move, far more than we would imagine about ourselves.

'Sometimes I go to my Egyptian dance class straight from work, and I'm so tired. But by the time I leave I'm buzzing!', one woman told me, adding: 'It's partly to do with the atmosphere of an all-woman group and the fact that it's a very supportive, rather than competitive dance. It does create a bond between the women in the group. I get far more out of it than just an exercise, more than just a dance.' Another woman said: 'I get a strength and joy from dancing. It feeds me. I suppose it allows a part of me that isn't shown in other ways to come out. You feel your naturalness coming out, your sensuality.'

I have seen many women blossom through mastering Arabic dance, seen them carry themselves with new pride, even seen painfully shy women develop the confidence to get up and perform spontaneously for the rest of the group.

Women who have suffered from particular illnesses have told me that, when doctors' advice and prescribed drugs have failed to help them, they have managed, through dance, to heal themselves. One woman in her late forties who had an operation for two prolapsed discs was left feeling worse, rather than better, after leaving hospital: 'My specialist told me I wasn't going to get any better. But I proved him wrong. Dancing gave me an incentive to get well. It played a big role in my recovery.'

There is a deep, underlying assumption in Western culture that expressing oneself on the dance floor is strictly for the young. I have grown very fond of one woman who comes to my summer school, and whom I guess to be in her seventies. She is a delicate-looking woman with tightly permed white hair, but her apparent fragility belies a strong will, and so far no one has been able to discover her age. The first time she was asked, she replied in a quavering voice: 'Old enough to have a driving licence.' Later on, after supper and a couple of glasses of wine, someone else made a similar inquiry and she said, deadpan: 'Old enough to know better.' But at the performance party at the end of the course she surprised everyone. She entered wearing a sheer black overdress lined with vivid red and a scarlet sash round her hips. She moved across the floor with a secret smile on her face, totally absorbed in her dancing, and at the end there were beaming smiles as well as looks of astonishment as the other women gave her a vigorous round of applause.

And then there are voluptuous women who have come to terms with their unfashionable size by discovering a dance which doesn't exclude them, but on the contrary, enables them to feel good about themselves.

An aesthetic in which youth and slimness are the sole criteria of beauty should be questioned. But it is not easy to challenge a fashion which so many people have invested so much time and money in promoting. It is not in the interest of our beauty industry to be broad-minded. It is not in the interest of the fashion world to accept human diversity. A great deal rides on persuading women that they are overweight, that having a few wrinkles is unsightly, that their bodies are the 'wrong' shape or, worst of all, that they are too old to enjoy themselves without looking ridiculous. Pregnant women especially suffer from the feeling that there is something shameful or absurd about their bodies, and few would choose to get up on the dance floor at this time of their lives.

Nur Banu is an Italian-Egyptian dancer, a professional performer with her own small company. She had two children in her youth and had no desire to add to her family. Then, when she was in her thirties, she discovered that she was pregnant again: 'I had a show booked and planned. I couldn't cancel it. By the time we were due to go on tour I would be eight months pregnant. What to do? I lay and stared at the ceiling for a few days. Then I thought, Alright, I'll do it. Of course it was difficult. I did not give myself a big part in the show, but I had to do the solo dance, there was no one else who could do it. I had a beautiful costume, a long dress, I remember. It was hard. I had to summon up all my energy. But, you know, the response from the women in the audience was incredible! So many women, they would come backstage afterwards with tears in their eyes. They told me: "We always thought we looked ugly when we were pregnant. We always thought we had to hide ourselves before. Now we see that we can look beautiful."'

'As soon as we come out of our mother's belly we dance!', laughs Tunisian performer Leyla Haddad. 'It's part of our everyday life. In my country everyone encourages you, as soon as you can walk, as soon as you start listening to music. And there is not this, "She dances well, she doesn't dance well" attitude. You don't condemn people. Everyone wants you to dance, and they don't understand it when people don't. Because, you know, everyone is a dancer in their heart.'

Index

Further Reading

Guests of the Sheik by Elizabeth Warnock Fernea (Anchor Doubleday, New York 1969) is an absorbing book about everyday life in an Iraqi village in the 1950s.

A Street in Marrakech, also by Elizabeth Warnock Fernea (Anchor Doubleday, New York 1976), is a similarly entertaining account of Moroccan women's lives.

The Blindfold Horse by Shusha Guppy (Mandarin, London 1992) is a memoir of growing up in Iran in the 1940s.

The Harem Within by Fatima Mernissi (Bantam Books, London 1994) examines women's lives and expectations in Morocco.

An Ancient Egyptian Herbal by Lise Manniche (British Museum Publications, London 1989) gives a detailed account of body care at the time of the pharaohs.

Sexuality in Islam by Abdelwahab Bouhdiba (Saqi Books, London 1998; paperback) is an excellent book on a complex subject.

Women in Islam by Wiebke Walther (Markus Wiener, Princeton 1993) is a thorough survey of women's lives and traditions, past and present.

For those interested in poetry and literature:

An Anthology of Modern Arabic Verse (Oxford University Press, Oxford 1970).

The Ring of the Dove by Ibn Hazm, transl. A. J. Arberry (Luzac, London 1953).

Treasury of Arabic Love Poems, Quotations and Proverbs, ed. Farid Bitar (Hippocrene Books, New York 1996).

Tales from the Thousand and One Nights, transl. N. J. Dawood (Penguin, Harmondsworth 1973).

The Perfumed Garden by Shaykh Nefzawi, transl. Sir Richard F. Burton (Neville Spearman, London 1963).

There are numerous nineteenth-century travellers' accounts of women's lives in the Middle East and North Africa which, while now out of print, can be picked up in secondhand bookshops. Extracts from these, charting Western perceptions of Arab women a hundred years ago, can be found in *Veiled Half Truths* by Judy Mabro (Tauris, London 1991). One which has recently been reissued is *Embassy to Constantinople: The Travels of Lady Mary Wortley Montagu* (Century Hutchinson, London 1988). *Women as Portrayed in Orientalist Painting* by Lynne Thornton (ACR Poche Couleur, Paris 1994) is a dazzling feast of images of women in the Arab world. Illustrated throughout in colour, it is available in both hardback and paperback.

For those who are interested in delving more deeply into the subject of massage I recommend:

Massage for Total Relaxation by Nitya Lacroix (Dorling Kindersley, London 1991); *The Massage Book* by George Downing (Penguin, Harmondsworth 1992); and *The Book of Massage* (Ebury Press, London 1984).

For more detailed information on the therapeutic use of essential oils, see *Aromatherapy for Women* by Maggie Tisserand (Thorson's, London 1985); and *The Fragrant Pharmacy* by Valerie Ann Worwood (Bantam Books, London 1990).

A Natural History of the Senses by Diane Ackerman (Phoenix, London 1990) is a cornucopia of fascinating information.

Finally, for those interested in dance I modestly recommend my book *Serpent of the Nile: Women and Dance in the Arab World* (Saqi Books, London 1994; paperback).

Picture Credits